8-26

Healing
YOGA

D1066812

ALSO BY LOREN FISHMAN

WITH ELLEN SALTONSTALL

Yoga for Osteoporosis

Yoga for Arthritis

WITH CAROL ARDMAN

Yoga for Back Pain

Sciatica Solutions

Back Pain: How to Relieve Low Back Pain and Sciatica

WITH ALLEN WILKINS

Functional Electromyography

WITH ERIC SMALL

Yoga and Multiple Sclerosis

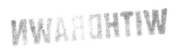
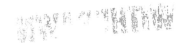

Healing

YOGA

Proven Postures
to Treat Twenty Common Ailments—
from Backache to Bone Loss,
Shoulder Pain to Bunions, and More

Loren Fishman, MD

W. W. NORTON & COMPANY

NEW YORK • LONDON

Author's note: The techniques described in this book, and the poses recommended for the reader, were carefully developed over the course of my many years in practice, and they reflect the methods that I have found effective in treating thousands of patients. No book, however, can replace the diagnostic expertise of a trusted physician who is familiar with your particular situation. Please consult a qualified medical professional (and, if you are pregnant, your obstetrician) before making any significant change in your exercise routine or if at any time you experience pain or nontrivial discomfort.

For information about permission to reproduce selections from this book, write to Permissions, W. W. Norton & Company, Inc., 500 Fifth Avenue, New York, NY 10110

For information about special discounts for bulk purchases, please contact W. W. Norton Special Sales at specialsales@wwnorton.com or 800-233-4830

Manufacturing by Courier Westford
Book design by Molly Heron
Production managers: Devon Zahn and Ruth Toda

Library of Congress Cataloging-in-Publication Data

Fishman, Loren.
Healing yoga : proven postures to treat twenty common ailments; from backache to bone loss, shoulder pain to bunions, and more / Loren Fishman, MD. — First edition.
pages cm
Includes bibliographical references and index.
ISBN 978-0-393-07800-8 (pbk.)
1. Hatha yoga—Therapeutic use. 2. Healing. I. Title.
RM727.Y64F57 2015
613.7'046—dc23

2014032915

W. W. Norton & Company, Inc., 500 Fifth Avenue, New York, N.Y. 10110
www.wwnorton.com

W. W. Norton & Company Ltd., Castle House, 75/76 Wells Street,
London W1T 3QT

1 2 3 4 5 6 7 8 9 0

FOR CAROL

my best friend,
first and last lover
and greatest teacher.

Contents

Healing
YOGA

Introduction

Is Yoga for You?

MAN, WOMAN, CHILD, senior citizen: the answer is yes. Novice, expert, teacher: the answer is yes. In good, medium, poor physical condition and fitness: yes. In my opinion, yoga is for everyone. Yoga provides physical and mental strength, balance and flexibility. It improves coordination. It improves mood. It has been used for thousands of years to treat common (and uncommon) medical conditions. Yoga is convenient. You don't need special clothes or shoes. If you use equipment, it can be simple: an old belt, a book, a card table chair. Yoga is democratic. Because so many people all over the world regularly practice yoga, it's easy to find. And it's portable—you can do it almost anywhere: in the backyard, on a plane, in a chair. Also, yoga is inexpensive or free. If I sound like a yoga aficionado, that's because I am.

Yoga has snugly fit itself into all parts of our society. You can do it in the studio, in the gym or at home. It helps people in prison, those with cancer and other illnesses, those who have returned from war. People of all ages benefit from it. What an amazing thing! Theistic but nonsectarian, not a sport, not an art, not exactly a science or religion. I am convinced that if all the world did yoga, Earth would be more peaceful, if only because we would all be devoting part of each day to improving ourselves.

Choosing Your Yoga

The practice of yoga started thousands of years ago in India. It's a testament to yoga's usefulness, both physically and spiritually, that it has survived into the present day, and that it has grown and evolved exponentially in a process that is still going on. Think about it. When I was in my twenties and began doing yoga in India with my teacher, B. K. S. Iyengar, hardly anyone was doing it back home in the United States. It was thought of almost as a pastime of people who were a little ... eccentric.

Now more than 20 million Americans practice yoga. And since so many of us are doing it, there is an almost infinite variety and richness of yoga types, styles and hybrids to choose from. You can do it in the air, while sweating in extreme heat, while laughing, while lounging in a swimming pool. You can do yoga with your dog, your child, your lover. You can do it quickly or slowly, competitively or not, with an emphasis on alignment, on breathing, on movement, on meditation or chanting. Some mix yoga and Pilates or other bodywork. You can find strictly therapeutic yoga to help you with just about anything that ails you, from addiction to knee pain (more about that below). You can go to class and learn yoga there. You can download courses or buy instructional DVDs and teach yourself at home. And I have mentioned only a few of the thousands of possibilities!

If you are not already a practitioner, the choices can be daunting, so I will be bold in my recommendation to you. After practicing yoga for more than thirty years, I suggest that you try the yoga I learned in Pune, India, when I studied with B. K. S. Iyengar—the yoga and meditation I still practice every single morning without fail. For me, Iyengar yoga has become a way of life. It's profoundly deep and complex, yet elegant; it provokes my thought and helps keep my body healthy. Iyengar yoga is anatomically sophisticated and therapeutically oriented.

I admire Mr. Iyengar for plumbing yoga to its depths to help people with health problems both physical and mental. When I was with him in India, he concentrated on alignment, which brought out the balanced, classic beauty in the poses and had an almost immediate effect on my feeling of well-being. Mr. Iyengar did not expect his students to have cookie-cutter bodies. In the classes I took in the bungalow where he had his yoga studio across the street from his home in Pune, there were fat people and thin people, tall and short people, old and young. We were together in a room, six or seven of us, practicing in whatever temperature Pune had to offer that day. Mr. Iyengar recognized that everyone could not do every pose to its fullest and encouraged the use of modifications to allow people to progress at their own pace. He introduced blocks, straps and other props, which are immeasurably useful, especially for beginners and for people who are older or have medical conditions.

This is not to say that I believe other ways of practicing yoga aren't valuable or good—many are. But those who teach Mr. Iyengar's yoga have been through a rigorous training over a period of years. They are prepared to teach, knowing that it is possible to injure oneself doing yoga. If you can, I suggest that you take Iyengar classes until you have enough experience to begin doing yoga at home, on your own. No matter what type of yoga you decide to do, whether it turns out to be temporary or a lifelong practice, the benefits are significant.

Doing Your Yoga

In his book *Outliers*, Malcolm Gladwell posits that it takes about 10,000 hours to achieve mastery in a field. As a doctor, I have a medical practice. I go to the office and see patients every weekday from 8 am to 6 pm. I have kept this same routine and discipline for many years. The result of this constant reinforcement of my profession is that I feel I am a better doctor now than I was the day I graduated from medical school. I'm a better doctor than I was two years later and twenty years later. The more I practice the more proficient I feel I become, and I have completed Gladwell's 10,000 hours several times over. Certainly that maxim applies to yoga. In order to reap yoga's benefits, you must do it. The more regularly and seriously you do it, the more time you spend doing it (assuming you have a good teacher), the more mastery you will achieve. I understand that when a simple forward bend relieves a spasm in your back, making you feel better in just a few minutes, you may dust off your hands and think, Well, that's that. But for benefits in addition to the physical, for that all-important sense of emotional well-being, do yoga regularly. Practice it as if you can become a master. Your progress may be slow, but I have seen transformations take place in those who practice patiently and with dedication.

Yoga changed the life of one of my patients, a reverend who was so obese he was beginning to have serious medical problems. His back, knees and feet hurt. He sometimes had trouble breathing. He began slowly and agonizingly, doing very simple poses and doing them with many modifications. As time went on something happened, perhaps because of his teacher, Cathy Lilly. He became interested in doing the poses. He got better at doing them. His self-confidence increased. He felt motivated to lose weight. He practiced yoga at home, in my office and even in Central Park, where, though he was still very heavy, he had a photograph of himself taken doing a near-perfect Ardha Chandrasana pose. Everything came together for this nice person. Yoga actually changed his life. He lost weight, and the last I heard he had started jogging as well and was signed up for a marathon. It sounds like a miracle. Maybe it *was* a miracle, but even if it was, this man's transformation began with yoga.

Yoga and Medical Science

When attending an International Association of Yoga meeting a while ago, I listened to Karen Sherman present her recently published clinical trial on yoga and back pain. That study got a tremendous amount of attention, and rightly so. It used rigorous Western standards to measure the efficacy of yoga and of ordinary stretching for treating lower back pain. It took Karen years to put together the model for the study and to bring it to fruition with participants. As I passed her in the hall after the meeting, I told her I was contemplating this book and asked if she had any suggestions. "Yes, I do," she said. "Please address the question of studying yoga with Western methods."

What is science? I immediately thought. What is "yogic" science? What, if anything, does the science we practice here in the United States—the science of double-blind, randomized, controlled clinical trials—have to do with the study of the chakras? How can we apply our Western standards to a science that didn't grow up in the same environment with them? Since all medical endeavors share a desire for results, one simple criterion for measuring the efficacy of yoga is: does it work? Controlled, double-blind, randomized studies work just as well for yoga as they do for toothpaste.

More deeply: if it is science, then there is a logical explanation for *why* something works, based on principles that are well supported. And that support is based on other principles, and so on back through thought and time.

This is true for all our beliefs. The magical substance thought to reside in wood to make it flammable gave way to Priestley's principle of oxidation. The ancient ideas about medicine and physiology have given up the spotlight to molecular biology and anatomy. But the ancient methods of objective comparison, and of reasoning through to a conclusion, are as crucial as ever. And although the means of proof have evolved, the benefits of the ancient practice of yoga have remained, and have already been demonstrated through application of modern statistical analysis and Western (really global) science.

Safe Yoga

A firestorm of concern, even outrage, arose when William Broad wrote in his book *The Science of Yoga* that people can "wreck their bodies" and seriously injure themselves doing yoga. While I have seen very few extremely serious injuries sustained while doing yoga, and while I believe with all my heart that yoga is for the most part safe, I know injuries can and do occur. The way to avoid injuring yourself is to choose a responsible teacher who has had at least two years of training, a teacher who asks if you have any previous injuries, one who watches as you do your poses to make sure that you are doing them correctly. If your teacher gives you a physical correction while you are doing a pose, make sure he or she is not forcing you. A teacher's hand should be light and gently guiding; it should never push, pull or shove. As I said before, props help people modify poses, making them less dangerous. If you feel extreme pain while doing a yoga pose, don't tough it out—just stop.

In this book I have given contraindications to each pose. Unless specifically indicated, these are relative, and the pose can be practiced with suitable props or modifications. Some such suggestions apply to everyone doing the pose. An example is Mr. Broad's and Mr. Iyengar's caveat: when doing the shoulder stand, always place a blanket under your head and neck.

Pre-Pose Points

When you're in pain or not feeling right, you're not able to do as much as when you're feeling fine, so begin slowly and carefully. Use the easier versions of the poses in this book and attempt to progress with judicious bravery.

1. If you master the pose and still have pain of any kind, carefully go forward to the more challenging version.
2. Alignment is of utmost importance, so pay attention to the classical poses' anatomical positioning.
3. There are good studies confirming the value and safety of many of the poses that follow. Others have not been adequately studied in the usual formal manner, but I have included them because I have observed their efficacy and relative harmlessness over many years of practice.
4. As you get better at yoga, yoga will be better to you, with more natural alignment and greater curative power.

Start out holding the poses for 10–20 seconds, and gradually build to a minute or more.

Repeated Poses, Relative Contraindications, Adaptations

Some poses are good for more than one problem and therefore appear in more than one chapter here. Ardha Matsyendrasana is an example—I've used it for both facet syndrome and piriformis syndrome. I have repeated these poses so the reader does not have to look up instructions from one chapter to another. Sometimes, however, I have adjusted the introductory sections: "Benefits," "How It Works" and "Contraindications."

If you are pregnant, talk to your obstetrician about doing yoga. Prenatal yoga is beloved by many, but each person and each pregnancy is different, so I recommend proceeding with caution.

Last, while I have given many variations and adaptations for classical poses in these pages (all variations are not pictured), I believe that resourceful practitioners will invent adaptations if they help.

The Scope of This Book

The information covered in these pages reflects the discoveries and adaptations I have made in three decades of practice. I believe they are all useful, but are nowhere near a complete encyclopedia of how yoga helps people— nor, certainly, the last word on the few topics that are discussed.

Nearly half this book is devoted to the different causes of back pain and how yoga can be used to treat them. Back pain is America's second most common ailment, just behind the common cold, and is frequently misunderstood. Almost every one of us has already or will in the future experience back pain. According to the American Academy of Pain Medicine, back pain cost employers an estimated $7.5 billion in 2011. Like the common cold (I'll get to that in a minute), some musculoskeletal back pain is transient. It disappears on its own in a relatively short period of time, or it may be helped to pass more quickly if the patient does the correct yoga.

Often neglected in the treatment of back pain, and what can make it a topic that is seven times larger than it would seem to be, is that there are seven very different causes of back pain. Their treatments are diverse, sometimes even contradictory. Yet many physicians and even clinical trials lump all back pain together as if it were only one problem. Without knowing which of the seven types of back pain you are feeling, you have many fewer possibilities for relieving it. My mantra is: get a diagnosis. Without one, you cannot possibly embark on a rational plan of treatment.

Back pain is one of my areas of expertise. I have had the privilege of carefully experimenting with various yoga poses for each of the seven major causes of backache and even finding ways to help patients who have pain with more than one cause.

The other common medical conditions I address in these pages may seem random, but they are widespread. The common cold strikes us all sometimes; over 40 million Americans have or are at risk for osteoporosis; an estimated 10 percent of Americans suffer from depression. Further, I have included conditions which researchers are studying to see how yoga might help. And then there are my pets: three conditions—restless legs syndrome, bunion and plantar fasciitis—that seem to me to be perfect for medical yoga. I know of no research yet on these conditions, but I have begun to do some research on them and I present my preliminary ideas here.

Yoga has not been studied for all medical conditions, nor is it necessarily appropriate for all medical conditions. I can only hope that scientists will continue to investigate the ways yoga works to help all sorts of medical problems. As time goes on, I believe research will provide enough information for at least one more book about the benefits of medical yoga.

PART 1

Back Pain: An Overview

E VERYONE GETS IT at one time or another. A child with a big backpack can get it; a person whose second home is his or her desk chair can get it; those who lug or lift groceries or other heavy things can be laid low. Back pain is the leading cause of disability in Americans under forty-five years old, according to one study that also found that more than 26 million Americans between the ages of twenty and sixty-four experience frequent back pain.[1]

Literally thousands of people with aching backs have trudged through my office seeking relief. Some of them are in excruciating pain. Once I saw a banker wearing a three-piece suit and newly shined shoes lying face down on the waiting room floor, a stack of MRIs near his elbow. Another of my patients, an aspiring actress, fell while waitressing, injuring her spine and leading her on a years-long quest for help, putting off her wish to start a family, perhaps permanently. I too have experienced back pain caused by a bulging disc. But often back pain—even back pain with a serious cause—eases by itself within weeks or months.

My mantra is, know the cause of your symptoms. If you have not identified the specific reason for your discomfort, you are unlikely to be able to treat it successfully. Back pain is a symptom, not a diagnosis. But a symptom of what? One symptom may have very different causes, as a man may limp due to arthritis or due to a stroke. Many of my patients who have practiced yoga with the goal of relieving back pain due to multiple causes have had amazing success. I can honestly say that yoga helps in almost every case. But at the same time, I have to caution everyone who wants to help himself or herself with asana (yoga postures): the diagnosis is everything. There is a reason for your symptoms, and I must emphasize that you need to find

11

out what that reason is. Yoga poses that cure one type of back pain might worsen an almost identical backache with a different cause. For instance, a forward bend may go a long way toward easing sciatica caused by spinal stenosis, but it could increase the pain or actually worsen a herniated disc.

As I am fond of saying, a person may have fleas or a person may have lice, or the person may have both fleas and lice at the same time. Don't discount the possibility that more than one problem exists in your back simultaneously. Still, when there are two or more problems, one is usually the main pain generator. The crucial thing is to identify the cause(s) and determine which one is contributing the most to your misery. In this book you will find a discussion and yoga poses both for self-diagnosis and for pain relief.

When to See a Doctor

I recommend you see your family physician or a specialist in rehabilitative medicine—my field—if your pain persists for more than ten days. If you lose bowel or bladder control, go to a hospital immediately. Your painful days are unlikely to reach into the double digits, but while you're waiting to feel better it makes sense to do certain things. The intelligent patient will observe the pain, identify it and quantify it. Where is it? When and how did it begin? Did something specific trigger it? Does it occur more at one time of day than another, more during one activity (such as sitting or driving) than another? How would you rate it on a scale of ten, where zero is no pain and ten is the worst possible screaming pain, and five is pain that intrudes on your concentration? What makes it better, even just a little bit? The answers to these questions are not just for your doctor. The more you know about your own condition, the more likely you are to be able to help yourself. The following sections will detail signs and symptoms you might recognize, and while you may not be able to diagnose yourself with complete accuracy, you can at least collect clues. If you do need to see your doctor, the information you have gathered will be valuable.

Neurological Pain

The first step in figuring out what's behind your back pain is determining whether the cause is musculoskeletal or neurological. This is almost always easy.

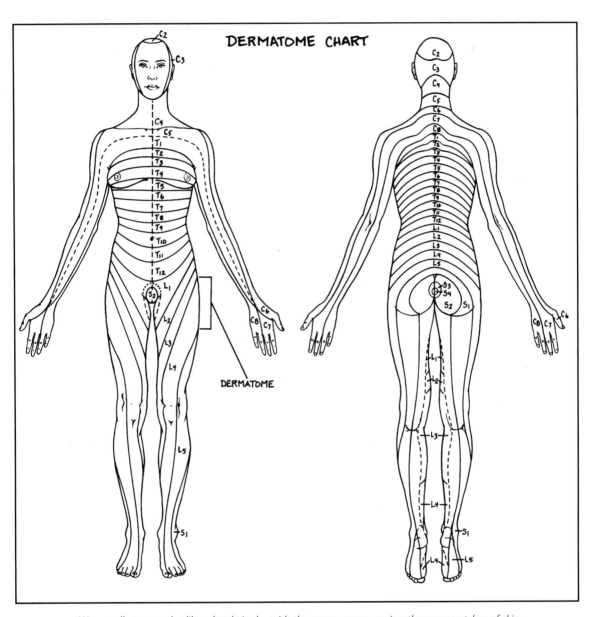

DERMATOME CHART

DERMATOME

We are all very much alike—hardwired—with the same nerves serving the same patches of skin and activating the same muscles, joints and bones. This fact can help you determine the neurological origins of lower back pain and other symptoms. Each numbered segment, or dermatome, corresponds with a spinal nerve root. So, for example, paraesthesias, numbness or pain in your outer calf indicate a problem at S1.

If you have numbness or weakness or pain going down your leg (even if pain occurs only in some places along your leg), then the odds are that your pain is neurological. The neurological causes of back pain are generally compression or irritation of the nerve fibers that travel down and exit the spine in the lower back.

Numbness, of course, is when you are unable to feel what is actually there: pressure, roughness, etc. There is an opposite condition, when you *do* feel things that are actually *not* there: tingling, pins and needles, hot and cold and other sensations that, like a mirage, don't actually exist. These feelings without an external cause are called paraesthesias. Their cause is almost always neurological.

It could also be that situation where there are both fleas and lice. So the next step is to determine whether symptoms appear elsewhere—say, in your arm or on the other side of your body. One part of your leg may be numb, while you experience a sensation of pins and needles in another area, perhaps your foot. Neurological symptoms ultimately have non-neurological causes. If you have severe arthritis which compresses nerve roots (this is not unusual), you may experience weakness. In some cases, the pain may be neurological but have nothing to do with your spine. You may become numb or experience paraesthesias due to a diabetic neuropathy.

Almost all the symptoms I've described appear along the course of the sciatic nerve. They're frequently lumped together by doctors and others under the category of sciatica, even though sciatica is not a disease; it's a symptom. Itching is also a symptom. Just as itching can be caused by poison ivy or chicken pox, conditions with very different treatments, sciatica can be due to dramatically different causes with dramatically different, even opposite, cures. When different kinds of back pain are lumped together under the umbrella of sciatica, the chances for relief are sharply diminished. As I said above but must repeat, if you try to treat the general symptom "low back pain" or "sciatica," you will often fail and may even injure yourself. In order to succeed, you must treat the thing that is causing the sciatica.

Sciatica

Sciatica—unpleasant sensations, from mild to intense, shooting down the back or side of one or both legs—is a symptom of something wrong in the back or buttock that is compressing or inflaming the sciatic nerve. The problem may also be much further up your back, if the nerve fibers that eventually form the sciatic nerve are compressed or irritated there. Often sciatica is caused by a herniated disc, where discal material presses on the nerve roots and inflames those fibers, or by spondylolisthesis. This Greek word sounds like what it is: slippage of one vertebra on the one below it, either forward, back or to one side. Spinal stenosis, a narrowing of the spinal column, can also result in sciatica. Then there is piriformis syndrome—unexpected under the umbrella of back pain, since it originates in the buttock rather than the spine—which occurs when the sciatic nerve is compressed by the piriformis muscle. Because it causes sciatica, naïve clinicians look for the source of pain in the lower back. To correct this limited view, I have included it in the section on back pain.

Of course sciatica can also result from an accident or (rarely) a tumor. You're more likely to develop sciatica if you lift heavy things or lift and twist at the same time, even with lighter weight. Sciatica may also result from poor posture, sitting too much, or a bullet wound.

Sometimes the pain goes down the front of the leg, following the course of the femoral nerve, which also originates in the back. That isn't sciatica, but it is the same thing involving another nerve. What is that thing? In thirty-five years of practicing medicine, I have yet to see a case that does not have a cause.

Musculoskeletal Pain

Problems in the muscles of your back, the alignment of spinal bones and other mechanical malfunctions account for a majority of the low back pain that afflicts just about everyone now and then. Musculoskeletal pain often goes away by itself before a couple of weeks have passed, but it depends on the details of your case: the exact reason for the pain, its severity, your physical condition and other medical problems. Sometimes, though you feel an improvement, lesser pain persists.

When the muscles and bones of the back get out of synchronization or alignment, the garden-variety backaches sprout and flower and sometimes become chronic. Pain can occur in the lower, middle or upper back. These backaches can be caused by bad physical habits, poor posture, repetitive motions, the stress of a fast-paced life or emotional problems. When you're hurting, you are likely to make adjustments in the way you sit, walk and even sleep. These adaptations to pain in one part of the back can cause more pain or discomfort in another part. If a sprain or chronic slouching causes discomfort in the lower back, the postural or other adaptations you make to get more comfortable may cause problems in your upper back. Your overworked muscles protest by clenching and going into spasm, which is extremely painful and can last for days or longer.

Muscle strain and spasm are two of the most common types of back pain. They are caused by heavy lifting, repeated bending and straightening and other vigorous activity, or by inactivity followed by forcible movement. When muscles are pushed to their limits or just beyond them, inflammation ensues, causing the muscle or group of muscles to contract strongly and to stay contracted in spasm, making it difficult even to get out of bed. Muscle spasms can be excruciating. They sometimes cause people to go to the emergency room, and doctors frequently prescribe muscle relaxants. But I think the best way to counteract a muscle spasm sensibly and sensitively is to stretch the muscle by doing yoga.

SPRAINS AND STRAINS

These words are often used interchangeably, but they have different meanings. According to the American Academy of Orthopaedic Surgeons, a sprain involves a ligament—the tough, fibrous, string-like tissue that attaches bone to bone.[2] When a ligament is overstretched or torn, the joint can be destabilized, causing pain. Spinal joints that are out of kilter can press on nerves, causing sciatica. A sprain can be mild, moderate or severe, and sometimes it's difficult to know if you have one. Indications to look for, besides pain, are bruising and swelling around the joint. In extreme cases, you may be aware of the wobble of an unstable joint.

A strain is an injury to tendons and/or muscles. Tendons attach muscles to bone. Overstretching of these tissues may also cause injuries that destabilize the spine. Strains and sprains can result from too much exertion, from lifting something heavy, from being overweight, taking a fall or a blow, even from a violent fit of coughing. People who jump in sports like basketball, or who engage in activities that twist or pull spinal muscles (sometimes to the point of tearing), can strain their backs. If that's what has happened, you may experience muscle spasm, weakness, swelling, cramping and in extreme cases an inability to move.

SPASM

When a muscle or a group of muscles in the back intensely contracts spontaneously and does not relax, you've got a spasm. Spasms often occur in muscles that are inflamed because of sports, pushing or pulling movements or sudden twists. Many back problems—arthritis, herniated disc and stenosis, to name a few—can contribute to the occurrence of a spasm. Postural problems, weak stomach muscles, weak or stiff muscles in the back and tight hamstrings are also common causes of spasm. Spasm is often underrated by the medical community: imaging studies are not conclusive, and blood tests seldom reveal a cause. But spasm is an unwelcome companion in many people's lives, and yoga is a simple and effective remedy.

Prevention of Back Pain

Though back pain strikes about a quarter of all adults for at least a day in every three-month period, there are tools that can be used for prevention, according to the National Institutes of Health.[3]

I believe a person who follows a regular yoga practice is less likely to have back pain than someone who doesn't, but as of this writing there are no large longitudinal studies that confirm this. What can be confirmed is that yoga increases strength, coordination, range of motion, reaction time, postural awareness and balance. It decreases anxiety. All of these benefits protect the back. Many of my patients who have back pain are afraid to exercise, afraid to move much at all. They're not babies, but the pain makes them baby their backs. The immobility increases stiffness and weakness and delays healing. Don't take to your bed if you have back pain. My advice is to rest if you need to, but also to move around a little, say about 40 percent of what you normally would do, and much more carefully—but *do* move, *do* stretch.

Standard Exercises for Simple Backache

The National Institutes of Health recommend four types of exercise for musculoskeletal backache, and I heartily endorse them. The first two, flexion and extension, involve stretching and occur in many yoga poses. Of course, physical yoga is all about stretching; it lengthens the muscles and soft tissues of the trunk, the legs, the arms and the neck, which can work wonders for those who are stiff and increases range of motion. Plus, it feels great. I recommend other movement too, including aerobic exercise, such as brisk walking, if you're up to it, which whittles away at stiffness, fear and the depression that sometimes comes over people who have bad backs. Aerobic exercise is good for your heart and good for general well-being; I suggest 30 minutes, but you can break this down into segments, then build up to your goal. But please remember: low-impact exercise is the way to go if you have back pain. Running on pavement, tennis, squash and other field sports are not recommended. Don't do impact aerobic exercise if you have significant back pain, and consult your doctor before doing any aerobics.

The exercises above are analogous to the aspirin you would take for a headache. It may help, or it may be useless. I repeat: until you have a diagnosis, you are treating symptoms and you must do so tentatively. This is just the first thing to do—first aid. Approach these exercises just as you might put calamine lotion on an itch before determining its cause. Sometimes the itch—or the back pain—will vanish, and there will be no need to go further.

Flexion: Flexion is the process of bending. Bending forward, even if it hurts a little, helps back pain by getting you moving. When you flex, you create space between the vertebrae in your back and feel relief because the nerves have more room and are not squeezed as much or at all. When you put yourself in flexion, you stretch your spine and the muscles around it, and also the muscles around your hips. A forward bend also puts your abdominal muscles to use, strengthening them. I am one of the majority of physicians who believes a strong core supports the spine and helps keep it healthy.

Caution: If you think you have a herniated or bulging disc, do not do forward bends, especially if they cause more pain. If you have osteoporosis, always lie on the floor when stretching your legs; never do it from a sitting or standing position because it could cause a fracture.

Extension: Backward bends, leg lifts or raising your trunk while lying on the floor on your stomach are some extension exercises. They have a way of helping to reduce sciatica or pain that radiates out from its source to other parts of the body. Arching your back often minimizes radiating or referred pain that is due to a herniated disc. Extension also widens some spaces between vertebrae and strengthens the muscles near the spine.

Caution: Extension exercises are generally contraindicated in spinal stenosis and spondylolisthesis, and helpful with herniated disc.

NON-POSE TIP

Change your shoes often.

Diagnose Yourself with Yoga

The suggestions below are not intended to substitute for a doctor's diagnosis and treatment. If your symptoms persist for more than two weeks, I suggest going to a rehabilitative medicine practitioner or to an orthopedist, neurologist or rheumatologist who can give you a definite diagnosis. In many cases, however, it is possible to get at least an idea of what's wrong by doing some yoga on your own. Again, I emphasize the importance of being careful. Be tentative. Don't push too much. I have developed these tests by trial and error, over years, and with the help of countless patients who have generously allowed me to try out my ideas while treating them.

- If forward bends help, you may have spinal stenosis; if flexion hurts, it suggests herniated disc or sacroiliac joint derangement. Exceptions: In a small number of cases, if the herniated disc is central—that is, in the middle of the spinal canal—or is broken off from the main disc mass, forward bends help and back bends hurt.
- If twists to one side help, and twists to the other side hurt, it suggests a herniated disc on the side to which turning is more painful.
- If back bends help, it suggests a bulging or herniated disc; if they hurt, your problem is more likely to be spinal stenosis or spondylolisthesis.

Nerve Root Symptoms Chart

Level of Problem	Pain	Numbness	Weakness	Atrophy	Reflexes
L₂-L₃ level 2nd lumbar nerve root	Lower back	Front and/or side of thigh	Weakness raising thigh with bent knee	Atrophy at inner thigh	Reduced reflex bringing thighs together
L₃-L₄ level 3rd lumbar nerve root	Lower back, any part of knee joint	Skin around knee-cap	Quadriceps	Quadriceps	Knee jerk diminished or absent
L₄-L₅ level 4th or 5th lumbar root	Buttock; outer and upper calf	Inner calf and instep	Weakness flexing foot upwards	Shin muscles below knee	Reduced reflex at front of ankle; no reliable reflex test
L₅-S₁ level 5th lumbar nerve root	Upper sacro-iliac joint, hip, outer calf and leg	Outer calf; skin between great toe and second toe	Weakness pointing foot	Inner calf muscles	Ankle jerk diminished or absent
S₁-S₂ level 1st sacral nerve root	Lower sacro-iliac joint, hip, outer thigh and leg	Back of calf; little toe, side of foot and ankle	Weakness of curling toes	Buttocks; back of calf and muscles of sole of foot	Ankle jerk diminished or absent

after Netter

Nearly invariable motor and sensory functions of lumbar spinal nerve roots are an invaluable guide for locating the causes of paraesthesias, numbness, pain and weakness.

But—and this may seem complicated—if the stenosis is due to a disc that is bulging into the spinal canal itself or a loose fragment, back bends hurt and forward bends may help. This occurs about 5 percent of the time, in my experience. That may not sound like a significant number, but if you are one of the 5 percent it is important. Be careful; don't push. It you feel worse, stop and try the opposite.

Since we are all hardwired identically (with very rare exceptions), the body itself is a virtual map of injuries. Nerve fibers from each level of the spine activate the same muscles in all of us, and weakness or lost reflexes in those muscles indicate the level of the problem quite precisely. For example, if you have weakness walking on your heels, it's the anterior tibialis that is weak, and the problem is at L4 (see chart on page 20). If your Achilles tendon reflex is robust on the right and absent on the left, most likely the problem is at the left L5 or S1, as the chart indicates. Numbness, paraesthesias and/or patches of pain in the front of the thigh? That will be L3.

Other Simple Diagnostic Maneuvers

SPASM

Spasm may occur anywhere: in the calf, in the quadriceps, in the large or small muscles of the back. The best way to assess this is to compare the tightness and tenderness of the muscle on the painful side with the same muscle on the opposite side. When you stretch a muscle in spasm, two things happen: at first, it hurts even more, but as you keep stretching, the pain almost invariably subsides below the level it was at when you started stretching. This is due to what might be called an engineering defect: muscles need supplies and services when they are working, but when they're working they contract, actually narrowing the capillaries that bring the blood which supplies oxygen, glucose and proteins to the muscle and carries away the toxic products of muscle metabolism. Usually the body handles this dilemma by alternating which little muscle fibers are active, a cerebellar process called rate coding. But in spasm all the fibers are active at once, and as the capillaries supply less blood, toxic substances such as lactic acid build up and irritate the muscle fibers, causing them to contract more tightly. The direct effect of this is to narrow the capillaries even further, reducing the blood supply even more—and we're off on a vicious and painful cycle. Stretching the muscle reverses all this, although at first you must overcome the force of the contracted muscle, which may not be an easy matter.

Feel the place where the problem seems to be, or get someone to lend a hand if you can't reach it yourself. The muscle will feel harder on the painful side than on the other side, and the hardness will follow the outline of the muscle. When pressed, a muscle in spasm hurts more, with a steady soreness. Pure spasm has none of the numbness or tingling associated with neurological problems. The only trick is to know your anatomy well enough to know which muscle is hurting, and how to stretch it.

NEUROLOGICAL PROBLEM AT L4 OR L5

Lie on your back with a belt at hand. Loop the belt around the arch of one foot, straighten the knee and raise it as high as makes sense for you. Then do the same with the other leg. If it just hurts behind your knees, that's normal, but if it hurts in the back, your problem is probably neurological and most likely at L4 or L5. This test, called the straight leg raise, is an even stronger indicator if raising the right leg causes left-side back pain (the contralateral straight leg raise).

SACROILIAC JOINT DERANGEMENT

Place a towel on a sturdy table and lie on top of it on your back. Cautiously sidle over to one edge, going far enough so your entire right buttock and leg are off the table. To avoid falling off—a genuine possibility—grasp the opposite edge of the table with your left hand. Now let your right leg slowly drop down toward the floor. If you feel pain in the small of your back or down in the sacroiliac joint(s) below the waist, above the tailbone and an inch or two to either side of the lowest part of the spine, it's a significant indication of sacroiliac joint derangement, though not an incontrovertible one. Be sure to test the opposite side to see which side feels more painful.

If there is numbness or weakness or tingling, then the problem is not sacroiliac joint derangement. It is very likely neurological.

PART 2

Musculoskeletal Back Pain

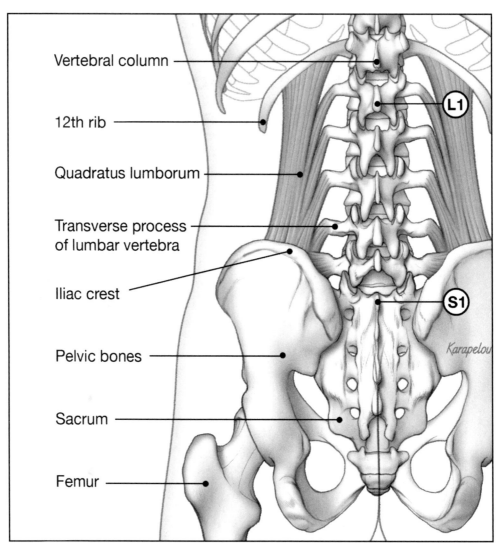

Vertebral column

12th rib

Quadratus lumborum

Transverse process
of lumbar vertebra

Iliac crest

Pelvic bones

Sacrum

Femur

L1

S1

Karapelou

The strands of the quadratus lumborum support the spine similar to the way cables support a tall radio antenna.

CHAPTER ONE

Quadratus Lumborum

Patients often come to me with the quadratus lumborum in spasm. Though you may never have heard the name of this powerful group of muscles, they are crucial in that they attach the pelvis to the spine by way of the ribs, and serve us by helping us bend our trunks from side to side. They also stabilize the lower back. When you're sitting at your computer, for instance, these muscles are working hard to keep your back steady and to keep your pelvis and spine in the correct alignment. However, they tend to go into spasm under certain conditions. Extreme bending or twisting or sitting for too long can push these hard workers over the edge, make them clench and cause severe pain. Here are some suggested antidotes.

Adho Mukha Virasana
Child Pose

Benefits and How It Works: Restful, stretches the quadratus lumborum muscles, countering spasm, stiffness or tightness. Increases your awareness of the muscles themselves, helping you gain control over them and encouraging them to relax.

Contraindications: Severe kyphosis, osteoporosis (use pillows under the chest in each of these cases), severely osteoarthritic knees (sit on blocks or pillows).

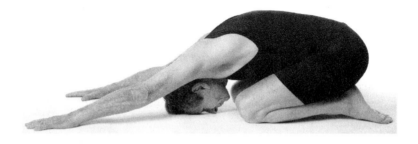

The Pose: Kneel and sit back on your haunches, placing a pillow over your calves or a block between your shins if necessary. Straighten your spine—get as tall as possible while making sure you are securely on your "sit-bones." Slide your palms forward against the floor until your torso reaches your thighs. Draw your shoulderblades back, together and downward toward your waist. Let your palms slide further beyond your head. Rest your head on the floor or on a block.

Ardha Baddha Padma Janusirsasana
Half Lotus Head to Knee Pose

Benefits and How It Works: Smoothly and naturally divides and conquers the hamstring tightness and quadriceps tightness that often accompanies quadratus lumborum spasm. The pressure of the lotus foot on the abdomen, and the forward pull of the arms and abdominal muscles create agonist–antagonist

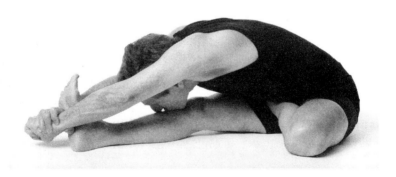

reflexes that will calm and stretch the very tough quadratus lumborum muscles. (An easy example of agonist–antagonist reflex is in the arm: when the biceps bends the elbow, the triceps, which straightens the elbow, simultaneously relaxes. This reflex applies to each pair of muscles with opposite function: contraction of one causes its antagonist to loosen.)

Contraindications: Osteoporosis, colostomy or recent abdominal surgery, concurrent herniated disc, severe knee or hip arthritis or replacement, sprained ankle, late pregnancy.

Helpful Hints: The straighter the leg and the higher the lotus foot, the better. It is better to go forward less far with a straight leg than to bend it, even if it means not appearing to stretch as much. If the leg is truly straight, inhibitory reflexes are activated that relax the hamstrings after 30–60 seconds.

The Pose: Sit with your right leg stretched straight out before you. Inhale, then exhale as you bend your left knee and place your left heel high against your right lower abdomen. Keeping your back straight, bring your torso forward. Hold your right foot, or clasp your left wrist with your right hand beyond it. Coax your chest forward, not down. Exhale and relax your elbows.

LESS CHALLENGING VARIATION:
Loop a belt around the sole of your foot. Remember to keep your back straight. Creep your hands forward along the belt until your elbows are straight. Aim the navel toward the inner front of the right thigh, rather than aiming your head toward your knee.

Parighasana
Gate Pose

Benefits and How It Works: This asana stretches the lateral fibers of the quadratus lumborum quite vigorously, and gives a gentler but more powerful stretch to muscle fibers closer to the midline, including the paraspinal muscles. It also works to lengthen the latissimus dorsi. This pose not only focuses on stretching one of these powerful, paired muscles at a time, it also varies the leverage on the outside fibers versus those located more centrally.

Contraindications: Prepatellar bursitis, vertebral compression fracture, severe facet arthritis, ankylosing spondylitis. Reduce intensity during pregnancy.

The Pose: Kneel with your knees together, pelvis tipped neither forward nor back. Lift your arms out horizontally. Take a few calm breaths. Straighten the right leg out to the side, heel on the floor and foot pointed upward. Align the right heel with the left knee. Slide the right hand, palm upward, out along the leg toward the ankle. Rest your head on your right arm. Raise your left arm overhead and press the back of your left hand into your right palm, or come as close to it as you possibly can. Except for the left shin and foot, your whole body should be in one plane. If your back arches, tuck your pelvis under. Repeat, switching sides.

LESS CHALLENGING VARIATIONS:

1. After kneeling, make a right angle with the right knee out to the side or proceed with straight right leg, as above. Rest your right forearm, palm upward, on your thigh. Incline to the right as much as is comfortable, raising the left arm, palm up, overhead and to the right.

2. Kneel, as above, with a chair facing your right side. Extend your right leg under the chair as you inhale. Exhale and grasp the chair back with your right hand, bracing your right forearm or elbow against the chair seat. Arch your left side, led by your left arm and hand to the right, palm facing upward. Breathe quietly for 20 seconds or so, then return to the central kneeling position, reposition the chair to face your left leg, and repeat the pose.

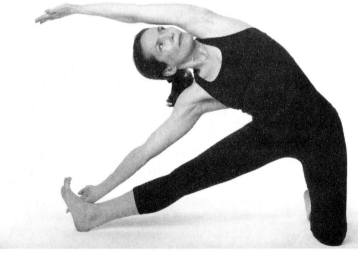

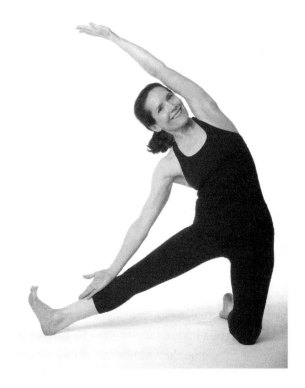

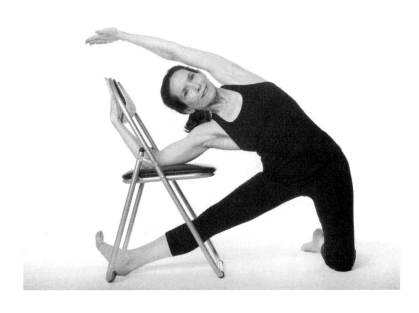

CHAPTER TWO

Tight Hamstrings

ANOTHER COMMON CAUSE of low back pain is stiff, shortened muscles in the backs of the thighs. The hamstrings stretch from the bottom of your buttocks to below your knees. Their job is to extend the hip joints and flex the knees. If they're tight, they limit your ability to swing your legs forward when you walk, prompting you to inch your pubic bones forward, tilt your pelvis back, and slouch.

Some of us inherit short hamstrings from our parents and are generally less flexible than other people. Or, bones may grow faster than muscles during the growth spurt that takes place around puberty, resulting in tight hamstrings that can be worked with but will always remain difficult. Even for those of us blessed with loose muscles, the culture can have a negative effect. Our desk habits and even our athletics favor contracting those muscles rather than stretching them. Sitting too much at a desk or in front of the TV allows the hamstrings to languish, stiffen and shorten, while many sports excite the muscle fibers, which then contract. That sitting, then immediately after being sedentary moving vigorously, can be a double whammy, straining already shortened muscles, prompting you to baby them, which tends to allow them to shorten and stiffen still further. A great many people, both those who are athletic and those who aren't, have shortened muscles in the backs of their thighs, making it difficult or impossible to bend over far enough to touch their toes.

The connection between shortened muscles in the backs of your thighs and low back pain may seem tenuous. But because of their effect on posture, tight hamstrings are one of the primary causes of aching backs. The pulling on the lower back muscles can also make joints slip out of kilter. Low back pain that results from tight hamstrings doesn't involve neurological symptoms—no numbness or tingling (unless a disc becomes herniated). But if bending forward hurts the backs of your thighs, you are more vulnerable to back pain than if you can touch easily your toes without bending your knees. Regular yogic stretching will help with posture and with comfort, and will reduce the potential for back pain.

Dandasana
Staff Pose

Benefits and How It Works: A number of people are so fearful of stretching their tight hamstrings it almost qualifies as a phobia. By assuming a familiar position everyone has assumed many times, this pose helps those who dread stretching to begin the process without fear.

Contraindications: Sprained hamstrings, ischial bursitis.

The Pose: Sit on a blanket or mat. Stretch your legs out in front of you, with your spine straight. Press your palms down on the floor, fingers pointing

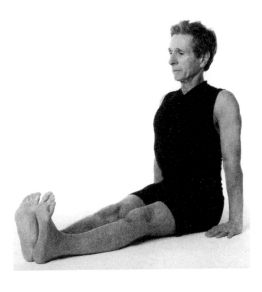

straight ahead, parallel to your legs and to each other. Even if you are facing a wall, look out to the horizon as you take a full, easy breath.

LESS CHALLENGING VARIATIONS:

1. If your hamstrings or other muscles crossing the knees and hips are too tight, the easiest way to start the pose is to incline your torso back and use your arms as support behind you. Point your toes. Then little by little come up toward vertical. Other postures in this chapter, such as Janusirsasana and Supta Padangusthasana I, below, should speed the process.

2. This is the easiest variation. Lie on the floor and walk your feet up a wall, straightening your knees with each step. Start far from the wall, walking up a reasonable amount and then sliding your heel up further to straighten your knee. When this is fairly easy and not very painful, move in a little closer to the wall. Another, similar variation is to lie to the left side of a doorway and stretch your right leg straight out on the floor. Then place your left foot on the wall just beside the doorway and gradually move it upward. After you can straighten the left leg, move further into the doorway and do it again. Then move to the right side of the doorway and repeat the procedure.

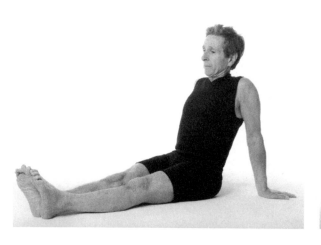 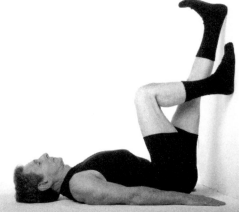

Trikonasana
Triangle Pose

Benefits and How It Works: A gentle and self-regulating way to stretch the hamstrings without injuring them. The reason it's self-regulating is that if you go down too far you start to lose your balance.

Contraindications: Severe plantar fasciitis, severe rotator cuff syndrome.

The Pose: Stand with your feet three feet apart. Turn the right foot out 90 degrees, the left foot inward 30 degrees. Stretch your arms out horizontally, and inhale. Exhale and incline the entire torso to the right, touching the floor beside your right foot. Don't allow your chest to turn toward the floor. Lower your right ribs to maintain a straight torso. Do not curve the torso, which will cause the left ribs to bulge out and upward. Place your hand on a block or on your shin if you are unable to reach the floor. Repeat, switching sides.

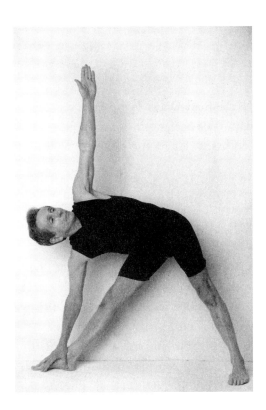

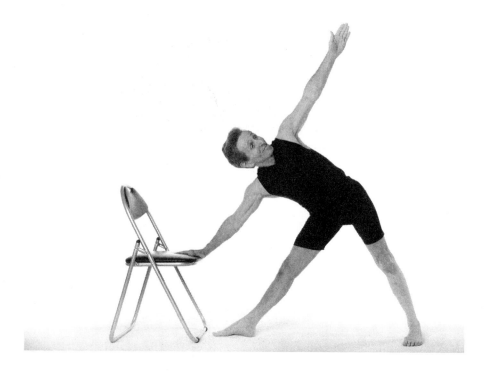

LESS CHALLENGING VARIATIONS:

1. Do the pose with your back against a wall.
2. Place a chair with seat facing the side you bend to. Rest your hand on the chair.

Janusirsasana
Head to Knee Pose

Benefits and How It Works: Stretches the hamstrings, one leg at a time.

Contraindications: Osteoporosis, herniated disc. The temptations to hunch the back are so great that if improperly done, this pose is a formula for compression fracture and acute herniated disc.

Helpful Hints: It is better to go forward less far with a straight leg than to bend it, even if it feels as if it is not stretching as much. If the leg is truly straight, inhibitory reflexes are activated that relax the hamstrings after 30–60 seconds, enabling greater stretch and initiating greater control.

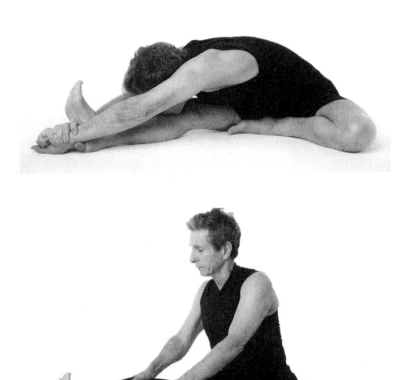

The Pose: Sit with right leg stretched straight out before you. Bend your left knee and place your left heel high against your right inner thigh. Keeping your back straight, bring your torso forward as you exhale. Hold your right foot, clasping your left wrist with your right hand. Coax your chest forward, not down. Relax your elbows. Take slow, even breaths. Repeat on the other side.

LESS CHALLENGING VARIATION:
Loop a belt around the sole of your foot. Remember to keep the back straight. Creep your hands forward along the belt until your elbows are straight. Aim the navel toward the front of the right thigh, rather than aiming your head toward your knee. Then relax your elbows. Let your elbows pull you down.

Supta Padangusthasana I
Reclining Hand to Big Toe Pose I

Benefits and How It Works: If there ever were a pose guaranteed to stretch the hamstrings, this is it. Pursue it vigorously, even passionately, but never too intensely. My experience with new practitioners is that it enlivens them; their faces become more integrated, more mobile, and appear more relaxed after Supta Padangusthasana I. The pose combines a number of effective mechanisms; it divides and conquers. By employing both arms to stretch one leg at a time, you can focus your efforts on a single set of hamstrings. Also, by lying on your back (*supta* is Sanskrit for supine) you protect delicate but stubborn structures from the minor to midsized forces that you may be tempted to apply to your tight muscles. It is safe in cases of osteoporosis, herniated disc and spinal stenosis. Third, the pose allows you to flex your quadriceps, which will have that agonist–antagonist reflex effect of relaxing your hamstrings. Last, you can bend the opposite knee, tilting the pelvis upward and giving you a better angle for stretching the straight leg. This won't help you make your hamstrings any longer, but will act as a safety valve to modulate how much of your effort goes into stretching.

Contraindications: Hamstring tear, severe congestive heart failure, late pregnancy (in which case it can be attempted, less forcibly, lying on either side), extreme hip arthritis.

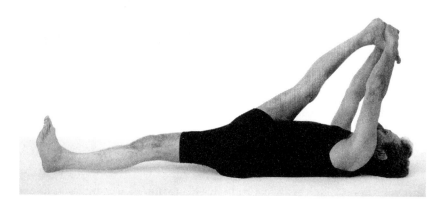

Helpful Hints: One of the reasons there are proportionately more injuries in men than women is that we males pit our greater strength against our lesser range of motion. I advise everyone to focus on relaxing the hamstrings rather than overpowering their resistance. When they resist, stretching them will hurt, causing them to resist more. If you concentrate on letting them go, they will stretch much more and hurt much less. Flexing the quadriceps is the key.

The Pose: Lie supine. Stretch out from the top of your head to your heels. Raise your right leg, grasping the ankle or foot with both hands. Exhale as you gradually lower your now straightened leg toward your torso, keeping both knees straight by contracting the quadriceps. Classically, the left leg stays horizontal as the right leg descends. When possible, adjust your hands' grip upward to straighten your elbows. Then the pulling downward will be done by the larger muscles of the shoulder and upper back. Breathe slowly and fully. Stay at least 30 seconds, then change sides and repeat.

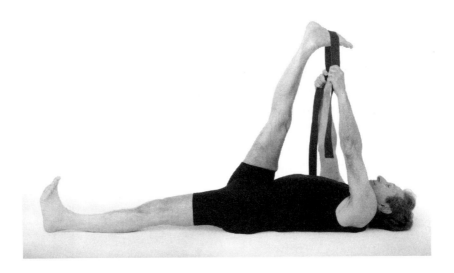

LESS CHALLENGING VARIATION:

A belt slung around the mid-foot is helpful at first. When using a belt, be sure to grip it high enough to bring the shoulders into play. Bending the opposite leg helps raise the straight leg high enough to get a better angle for the stretch.

CHAPTER THREE

Facet Syndrome

THE TINY SETS of joints that connect the vertebrae to one another are called facets. A major cause of back pain is facet joints that are out of kilter due to arthritis, unusual twisting activity or spasm. If a facet joint is responsible for the pain, the pain may radiate but you will not feel weakness or numbness or electric shocks. Some physicians, and I am one of them, believe that facet syndrome—pain because of a problem with the facet joints—can be due to tight muscles between two spinal segments beyond the joints themselves. In those cases, yoga stretches may be the perfect treatment. (See also chapter 5, "Herniated Disc," and chapter 6, "Stenosis.")

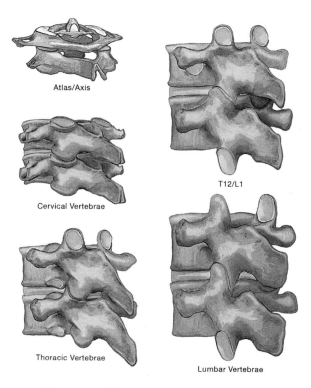

Atlas/Axis

Cervical Vertebrae

Thoracic Vertebrae

T12/L1

Lumbar Vertebrae

Facet joints differ according to their function.

38

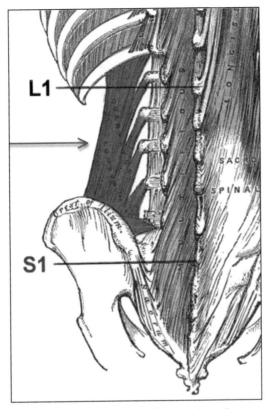

Tight muscles can cause "facet syndrome."

Supta Virasana
Supine Hero Pose

Benefits and How It Works: Trains the many intervertebral muscles to work together.

Contraindications: Hyperextension of the spine (lumbar lordosis), severe hip, knee or ankle arthritis or meniscal tears, recent abdominal or breast incision or hernia.

Helpful Hints: This is not about hyperextension but about getting the small of the back down to the floor. Many people need one or more blankets, or a bolster, under their backs. Please be very careful; ease yourself into the pose gently to protect your back.

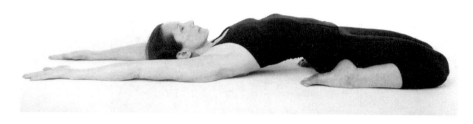

The Pose: Kneel and sit back so your buttocks are between your heels. If you need to, sit on a block. Take two breaths. Place your palms on the floor beside your feet. Recline by bending elbows until forearms are flat on the floor. Slide elbows forward until the shoulderblades are on the floor too. Raise both arms straight over your head, laying the backs of the arms and hands on the floor. Stretch from your fingernails to your kneecaps. Let your lower back descend to the floor, or to a blanket, a block or a bolster.

LESS CHALLENGING VARIATION:

To safely move the facets, grasp the ankles of a friend standing on tiptoes behind you, at a distance of the arms' complete stretch. The friend should

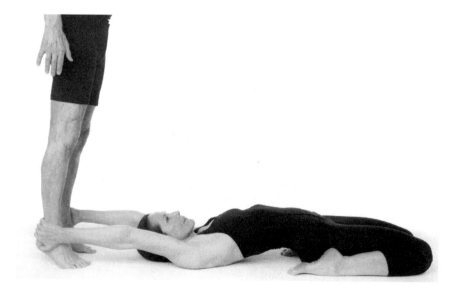

then gradually tiptoe backward, and when you have used that extra aid to stretch further, the friend should go down on his or her heels. Repeat the tiptoe-back-and-descend procedure within safe limits.

Marichyasana I
Forward Bend with One Bent Knee Pose

Benefits and How It Works: Separates upper from lower half of facet joints, enabling them to slide into the normal position. Stretches muscles that connect one vertebra to the next.

   Contraindications: Ischial bursitis, herniated disc, osteoporosis.

   The Pose: Sit with your right leg straight out in front of you. Bend your left knee so the shin is vertical. Wrap the left arm around the left shin high up near the knee, starting from the inside of the leg. Exhale and reach your right hand behind you until you are holding your left wrist. Take a breath. Exhale again, taking care to retain a straight back as you draw your torso forward with the left shoulder and elbow while pushing it forward with the back of your left upper arm. Breathe in and then exhale a third time as you descend symmetrically, bringing your sternum close to the inner right knee.

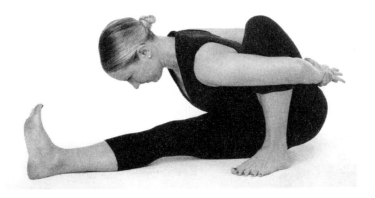

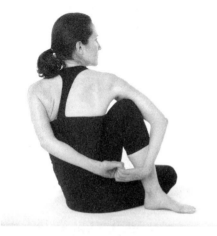

Matsyendrasana
Seated Twist Pose

Benefits and How It Works: Gives controlled opening to all the facets on one side of the spine, and stretches the paraspinal muscles at the same time.

Contraindications: Total hip prosthesis, anterior shoulder subluxation, severe scoliosis.

Helpful Hints: Attempt to keep your pelvis level. Breathe by inflating both lungs as equally as possible.

The Pose: Sit with your right knee bent to the left, its lateral thigh and calf on the floor. Bend and lift the left knee, then place your left sole flat on the floor to the right of the right thigh. Angle the outside of the right upper arm to the left of the left thigh as you revolve your torso to the left. Bend your right elbow as you reach counterclockwise behind with your left hand, eventually to clasp your right and your left hand. Keep your head level as you turn it to the right. Sit tall. Breathe symmetrically.

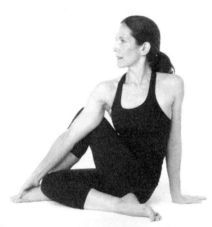

LESS CHALLENGING VARIATIONS:

1. Rather than bending your right elbow around your left shin, keep the right elbow straight. Press it firmly against the outside of the left knee and walk the left hand counterclockwise behind you.

2. Reverse your legs from the versions above. Place your right hand on the mat beside and behind your right thigh, keeping the elbow straight. Place your straightened

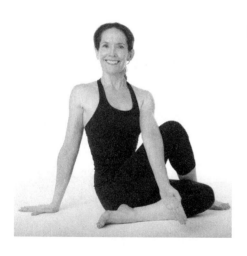

left arm to the right of your right thigh. Use the outside of the left thigh to lever the torso and twist somewhat less extremely and with more control to the right. Remember in both of these versions to sit straight and to revolve at the spine, not the sternum.

Supta Padangusthasana II
Reclining Hand to Big Toe Pose II

Benefits and How It Works: Subtly twists and bends the entire lumbar spine to the side in a controlled way, opening the facet joints and sliding their surfaces past one another.

Contraindications: Acute hamstring or adductor tear, advanced congestive heart failure, advanced pregnancy (in which case, elevate the leg vertically while lying on the opposite side).

The Pose: Lie on your back, heels together, shoulders down toward your hips, head far from shoulders. Raise your right leg and bend your knee in order to grasp your big toe with the index and middle fingers of the right hand. Straighten the right knee and stretch the leg off to the right at 90 degrees until it lies against the floor. Gradually separate the two legs even further by pulling the right leg toward your right. Stretch your left leg maximally, sliding your left heel away from you as much as possible. This stretch is vital for aiding the facets.

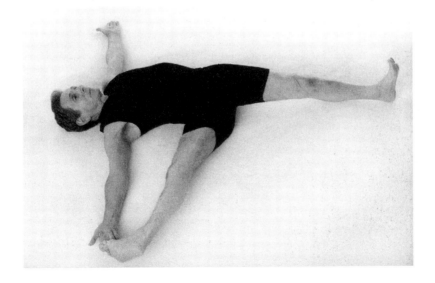

In each of the following variations, be sure to stretch the left heel out as far from the torso as possible.

LESS CHALLENGING VARIATIONS:
1. Loop a belt around the right foot.
2. Place a block for your foot to rest on when your leg goes out to the side.

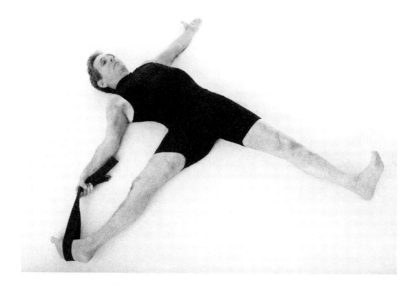

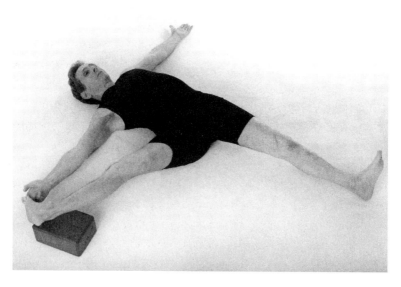

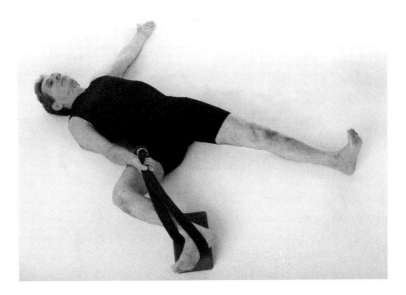

3. Keep the right knee slightly bent when moving it to the side.

Parivrtta Janusirsasana
Revolved Head to Knee Pose

Benefits and How It Works: Stretches interspinal muscles and moves the facet joints past one another, one side of the spine at a time. Most facet or intersegmental pain is in the thoracic spine. Using a twisting motion at the shoulder girdle together with iliopsoas muscles' stabilizing influence on the lumbar spine forcibly but gently stretches the interspinal muscles while sliding the facet joints smoothly, with room for compensation by the vertebrae above and below any painful and tender section.

Contraindications: Recently herniated disc, osteoporosis, severe scoliosis, adductor or hamstring tear, ischial bursitis, anterior shoulder subluxation, pregnancy.

The Pose: Begin by sitting in Janusirsasana, right leg stretched out before you, left knee bent, left foot flat against the upper inner right thigh. Take a breath. Abduct and extend the left hip, widening the gap between right and left thighs. Your left shin will no longer make a right angle with the right thigh; rather, it will make an obtuse angle of perhaps 135 degrees or more. Then incline your right torso forward, bending as much as possible from the hip, and angling your right elbow

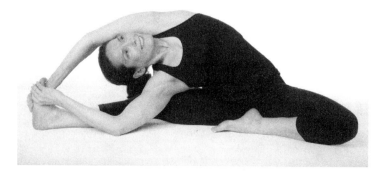

to the inside of your right knee. Externally rotate the arm to catch the right big toe with the little finger side of the right hand. Elongate your spine as you exhale.

Press the outside right elbow against the inner right knee to revolve your right torso forward and your left torso backward. Inhale, and as you reach forward and behind your left ear with your left hand toward the right foot, exhale. Finally, press your right elbow against the inner knee one more time, and with your next exhalation lengthen the spine still more and twist as much as makes sense for you.

You may hear or feel the vertebral facets clicking into place as you do this on one side or the other or both.

LESS CHALLENGING VARIATIONS:
Simple and sensible variations have less forward bending and less twisting. Use walls, chairs, belts and bolsters to fit your needs and capacities, and be cautiously creative with your modifications.

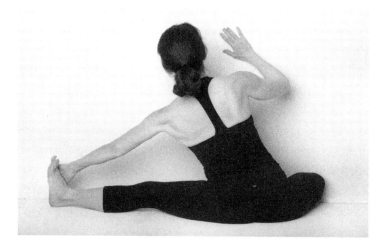

CHAPTER FOUR

Sacroiliac Joint Derangement

SACROILIAC JOINT (SI) derangement is perhaps the most under-recognized and untreated cause of low back pain. Some say 15 to 30 percent of individuals with chronic back pain that is not neurological and does not originate in the spine suffer from this problem, but I believe the percentage is higher.[1] In the past, a poor understanding of this condition, and the refusal by some medical professionals even to recognize its existence, made it difficult to get a diagnosis and successful treatment. Recently there has been more interest in this condition, partly because it is so painful, and partly because it can lead to other spasm and piriformis syndrome.[2]

You have two sacroiliac joints, one on each side of the midline sacrum a little below your waist. While other major weight-supporting joints—the knees and ankles—are flat and horizontal, the SI joints, which are in line with the kidneys, are vertical. Did nature make a mistake, giving us a central weight-supporting joint that is nearly vertical? If we walked on all fours, the sacroiliac joints would be horizontal and the forces these joints bear would be more evenly distributed. They would be less susceptible to injury. But in humans, who are upright and walk on two legs, their position and shape make them more vulnerable than other joints in the body. The sacroiliac joints support the heavy torso, arms and head, and hold us steady when we move and twist. That's a big burden for these structures, and because they do so much and bear so much weight, they need very strong ligaments to hold them in place. Yet they must be capable of adaptive movement. As I will explain below, these strong ligaments are two sides of a double-edged sword.

The SI joints are complex, three-dimensional bony junctions that have many irregular depressions and ridges. To function properly, everything must fit together perfectly, like the pieces in a complicated jigsaw puzzle or a key in a lock. The SI joint has a very small range of motion. In fact, its movement is measured in millimeters. When it moves out of alignment, the pain is terrific. Worse, when alignment is faulty, those strong ligaments that usually keep the joints in place play a negative role by holding the joint in misalignment, concentrating all the pressure usually spread across the entire joint on tiny, ill-fitting areas. Realignment is often gradual, despite the joints' small range of motion.

Nonsteroidal anti-inflammatory drugs (NSAIDs) can produce good results when used early, and because spasm often accompanies derangement, some physicians prescribe a muscle relaxant in the early stages of this condition. Physical therapy, chiropractic, osteopathy and anesthetic injections are sometimes used with greater or lesser success to treat SI joint problems. I have found yoga to be an excellent tool for repositioning the structures and for pain relief.

Diagnosing SI Derangement

If you have SI derangement, X-rays, MRIs and EMGS won't show any but the most egregious pathology. Still, you may be able to diagnose yourself. The pain is usually restricted to the small, specific area where the joints are, below your waist and about two inches from the midline. The pain can be on one or on both sides, but usually it is more intense on one side than the other. The pain can move from side to side. Unless there are complications, pain doesn't usually radiate down the leg, but it intensifies when you go from a sitting to a standing position. Exiting the back seat of a car can really hurt. The grinding or gnawing ache may get worse with certain movements, such as reaching up while standing, bending down while your knees are locked, or getting out of bed in the morning. Twisting to one side is likely to hurt more than twisting to the other side. Neurological symptoms such as weakness, numbness and tingling are absent unless the problem has become chronic (which it often does) and has caused you to make adjustments in the way you walk and stand—adjustments that create additional and possibly neurological problems. SI derangements are considered chronic if they last more than six months. SI derangement can be the result of an injury such as stepping into a pothole, but it can also come from having legs of different lengths, and pregnant women are susceptible. Pregnancy is a triple whammy because distribution of weight is changed, the placenta secretes the hormone relaxin, which loosens ligaments, and, late in the game, women sleep on their sides. If you have SI derangement, the sooner it is diagnosed and treated the better. The longer one or both sacroiliac joints are out of alignment, the more difficult it is to correct the situation.

Since the nineteenth century, movement and positional abnormalities of the sacroiliac joint have been documented, and treatments have been suggested.[3] Yet the condition continues to defy easy diagnosis and cure, and more research is certainly warranted. Nevertheless, I recommend a simple test for SI derangement. Lie flat on a table or other hard surface that is off the floor. Move one side of your body and one buttock off the edge. Using a wall or furniture for balance, to prevent a fall, let one leg hang over the edge. If that causes pain below the small of your back, you may have SI derangement. There are other tests, the best of which requires an experienced person to put their thumbs on your posterior superior iliac spines (PSISs) and assess if they move asymmetrically as you bend forward. If they do, and your legs are the same length, it's likely a sign of SI derangement. While the pain of SI derangement is always in the lower back, it's difficult for some people to pinpoint it. Some of my patients think mistakenly that the pain is in their hips.

Yoga for SI Derangement

SI derangement is relieved by yoga for several reasons, not the least of which is that it can be worked on little by little over time. Unlike a dislocation in another part of your body, say in your shoulder, the SI doesn't just slip back into place. The more usual course is physical therapy which causes the bones to move back into alignment little by little until the pain disappears.

Unlike physical therapy, chiropractic or osteopathy, yoga enables you to work on the problem at home, at your own pace. As you do, you are likely to reduce the tone and spasticity of the muscles around the joint. This will make them less likely to fix the joint in the wrong position. At the same time, yoga loosens nearby joints, relieving stress on the SI joint. This sharing of movement will help the SI joint itself if it is misaligned, and also help prevent reaggravating it. If the joint is out of alignment, yoga can open it and enable its constituent parts to move. Body awareness is a big benefit of the practice of yoga, and it is important when it comes to relieving pain and preventing it in the future. Yoga is also suitable for pregnant women, who are unable to take medications.

These poses can be done as often as you like, before or after meals, without any danger. In all three of these poses, you may hear a click or feel a pop as the sacrum slips closer to its true position, or you may hear and feel nothing. If the pose succeeds, you will feel better almost instantaneously, whether you've heard or felt something or not.

Gomukhasana
Cow Pose

Benefits and How It Works: This pose separates the lower parts of the pelvic bones from the sides of the sacrum, enabling the sacrum to readjust itself and

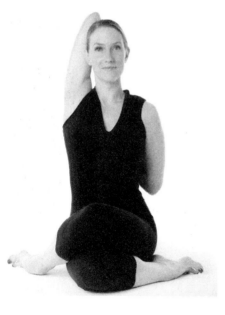

slip back into its proper position.

Contraindications: Total hip or knee replacement, trochanteric bursitis.

The Pose: Sit on a flat surface, right thigh directly in front of you, knee bent off to the left. Lift your left leg and carry it over to your right, aligning the knees straight in front of you. Raise your right hand over your head and drop the hand down your back. Extend your left hand behind you, and raise it. Clasp your left hand with the right. Straighten and lengthen your back, puff out your chest and gaze straight ahead.

VARIATIONS:

1. To make conditions more favorable, submerge yourself in a warm bath for five to ten minutes, and do the leg portion of the pose for a few minutes while you are in the tub. Then stretch out on your back in the bathtub for another five to ten minutes. Submerge to your jawbone.

2. If it's difficult to align the knees straight in front of you, press your palms against the outsides of the thighs to approximate alignment as best you can. Straighten and lengthen your back, puff out your chest and gaze straight ahead.

3. If you have rotator cuff syndrome or frozen shoulder, do just the leg portion of the pose.

Garudasana
Eagle Pose

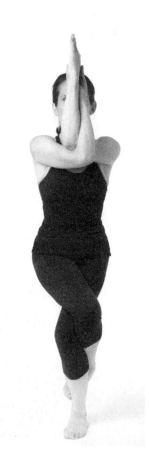

Benefits and How It Works: This pose separates the lower parts of the pelvic bones from the sides of the sacrum, as you tighten the pose by squeezing one ankle against the opposite calf. The sacrum can then readjust itself and fit back into its proper position.

Contraindications: Do not do this pose if you have had a total hip replacement. Do it carefully or not at all if you have had a total knee replacement or a medial or lateral meniscal tear.

The Pose: Sit on a chair, cross your right leg over your left and hook your right ankle behind your left calf. Place your left upper arm in the crook of your bent right elbow; orient your palms vertically, place them together and raise them to eye level. Elongate your spine. The classical version of the pose has you standing, but you can remain seated if getting up is painful. Then repeat the pose with the other leg on top, the other arm giving the support.

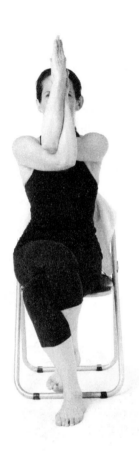

VARIATION:

Place your palms on your thighs and push your torso gently upward as you inhale. Even though one thigh is above the other, make the pressure symmetrical. As in Gomukhasana, the legs-only version may be more helpful than the classical pose. By lifting all the structures that press down on the sacrum, this version enables the sacrum and iliac bones to regain equilibrium and return to their anatomical alignment.

Mayurasana
Peacock Pose, a distant variation

I call this pose "Leaning," and many of my patients find it extremely helpful.

Benefits and How It Works: Uses gravity to pull down the iliac bones while the sacrum, spine and all higher parts of the body are being held up. This applies some force to separating the sacrum from the iliac bones and lifting up and away. This pose reduces the downward force that gravity exerts on the joint itself, permitting the sacrum to recenter itself between the iliac bones, thus reestablishing proper alignment and movement.

Contraindications: Carpal tunnel syndrome, severe osteoporosis.

The Pose: Stand facing a table or between two chair backs. Place your palms, facing forward, against the edge of the table or on the chairs approximately as far apart as your shoulders. Bend your elbows and lean forward to press your lowest rib against your elbows at the table, or straighten them if you are using two chairs. Transfer some of your weight from your feet via your ribs to your elbows or your shoulders (with the chairs). Relax your abdominal muscles: front, sides and back. Take shallow breaths for 20–30 seconds.

VARIATION:

Sit in an armchair, as pictured, palms on the chair arms, forearms parallel to your torso. Lift your torso slightly. It is not necessary to actually raise your thighs off of the chair, just to lessen some of the gravitational force on them. This makes it easier to relax the abdominal muscles. Remember, the abdomen has front, sides and back: paraspinal muscles and quadratus lumborum in the back, latissimus dorsi on the sides. All must be relaxed if this pose is to work. This is not an athletic event; relax all the muscles, get a jelly belly.

In this modified pose you can slant to the right and left, forward and back, and twist to either side. You can therefore relieve the pressure on your sacroiliac joint in all three dimensions, and combine these motions, e.g., slanting to the right, leaning forward and twisting to the left. In this respect, it is the more versatile and useful version of the pose.

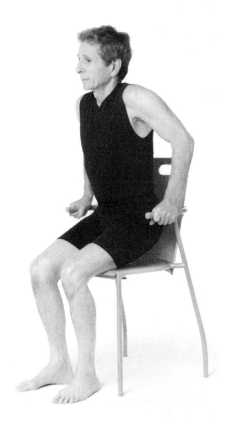

Relaxing the abdominal muscles is not easy for everyone. You'll know you are doing it correctly if you feel some stretching and a dull ache in the lower spine, just above where you feel the broad expanse of the iliac bones. You may have to experiment with this pose, whatever version you use. It may come easily, or it may take you a week or more to find the position that relieves your pain. Once you find it, the pain may recur in a matter of hours, and it may take more attempts to find the right position again. Over time, the solution will come to you faster and last longer.

PART 3

Neurological Back Pain

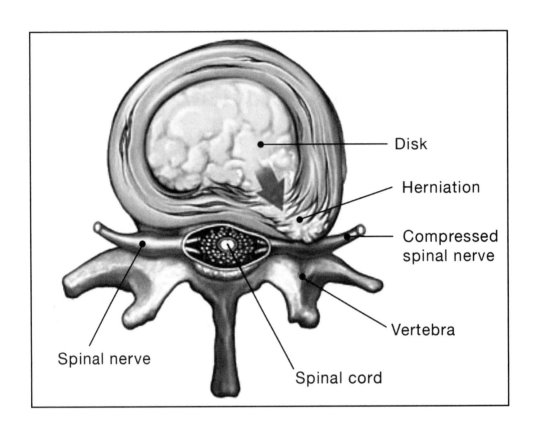

Disk

Herniation

Compressed
spinal nerve

Vertebra

Spinal nerve

Spinal cord

CHAPTER FIVE

Herniated Disc

THERE IS A widespread and warranted belief that much low back pain disappears by itself in time, including the pain of an intravertebral disc whose surface is cracked and has partially or completely leaked its contents—a disc that has become herniated or "slipped." Herniated discs can occur suddenly from an activity as innocent as bending down to pull up a small weed or from playing rough sports—a risk that is increased by the simple, inevitable process of growing older—or from an accident.[1]

This very common medical condition lays people low. It causes sciatica. It prompts doctor visits. The pain of a herniated disc can last a long time, sometimes years or decades, but studies have shown that people with severe back pain often return to work about two weeks after it begins. In one study, over 80 percent of people who had been laid up by back pain were working at the end of three months. Yet after a whole year, only 72 percent of participants in that clinical trial reported complete recovery from their pain.[2]

Only after years of using yoga in my medical practice did I dare to prescribe it for patients with a herniated disc, because it is such a serious cause of back pain and sciatica. The first time I tried yoga for this condition was with a stocky forty-five-year-old patient who worked in an auction house, moving fancy furniture, heavy paintings and old books. He was in a lot of pain and had already had epidural injections and physical therapy. His EMG and MRI showed a herniated disc, so his diagnosis wasn't in doubt, but by the time he came to see me he had a pretty severe aversion to the high-tech medical world and its treatments. As he was telling me that he didn't want any more tests or injections and he certainly didn't want surgery, it dawned on me that I could try him in a standing pose called Warrior I. He'd never done yoga, but almost as soon as he began he started giving me positive feedback about the way he was feeling. So I forged ahead.

After the standing pose, I asked him to lie on his stomach on an examining plinth. Then I showed him a gentle Locust pose. I told him when he got tired to lie down and rest and went to my desk to dictate a note. When I checked on him five minutes later he was still in the Locust! And he told me that it was the first time in four years he had been pain-free.

Of course, the process of healing took longer than one office visit, but that day gave him confidence and established the therapeutic alliance we needed for him to do the yoga diligently. During the next six weeks he practiced faithfully and got rid of his pain.

This success encouraged me to try other poses with other back pain patients until it has become almost routine. After some months and more and more patients doing yoga in my examining room, I decided to conduct a small therapeutic class. I didn't ask myself if other physicians were doing the same thing—using yoga regularly in their practices; I just fulfilled a dream that I hadn't exactly articulated or acknowledged even to myself. But it was a dream that had been lying fallow for many years, an intention I had had even before I went to medical school.

Pre-Pose Points for Herniated Disc

When you're in pain, you are not able to do as much, so start very cautiously, with less challenging versions of the poses. Pay attention to your alignment; it's crucial, and as you practice your body will adapt to the pose. Start out holding the poses for 10–20 seconds and gradually build to a minute or more.

Salabhasana
Locust Pose

Benefits and How It Works: Draws the herniated disc forward to align with the vertebrae and out of the region where it is irritating the nerve. Strengthens the muscles that do so.

Contraindications: GERD (gastric reflux), spinal stenosis, pregnancy.

The Pose: Lie face down, arms at your sides with your palms down. Stretch your body out from the top of your head to the bottoms of your heels. Lift from your Adam's apple and your hamstrings. With ankles together, inhale and lift your arms parallel to the floor, palms facing each other. Elongate your entire body.

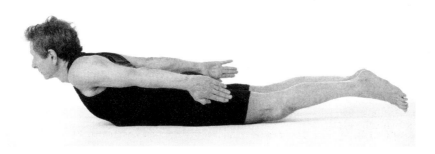

LESS CHALLENGING VARIATIONS:

1. Place your palms underneath your shoulders and press down to raise your torso. Most of the lift should come from your back muscles, not your arms.

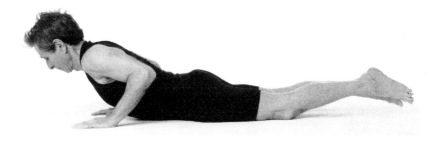

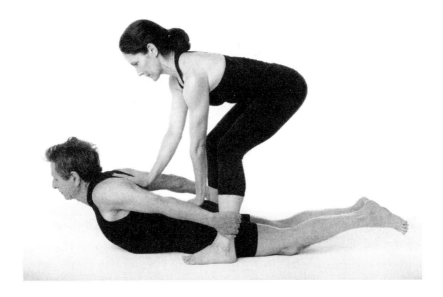

2. Hold the shins of a partner who straddles your torso, as shown.

MORE CHALLENGING VARIATIONS:
1. Interlock your fingers behind your head.
2. Stretch your arms out in front of you, or out to your sides airplane fashion.

Setu Bandhasana
Bridge Pose

Benefits and How It Works: Opens the chest, a postural improvement that relieves herniated disc pain and creates a more flexible, resilient cervical, thoracic and lumbar spine.

Contraindications: Herniated cervical disc, advanced arthritis, advanced pregnancy.

The Pose: Lie on your back with a folded blanket under your shoulders, but not under your neck or head. Bend your knees and place your feet on the floor. Push your feet away from you without moving them, using the force to lift your torso and pelvis. Support yourself with your hands under your lower back, elbows at right angles.

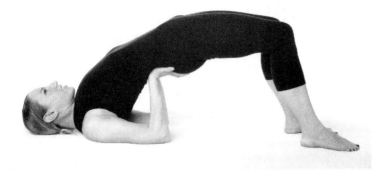

LESS CHALLENGING VARIATIONS:

1. Instead of lifting your torso, lie in a similar position on bolsters, large pillows or multiple blankets.

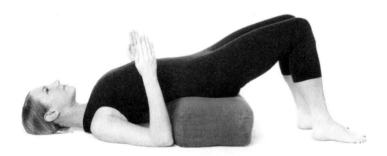

2. Place a bolster or a block underneath your sacrum and lift from there.

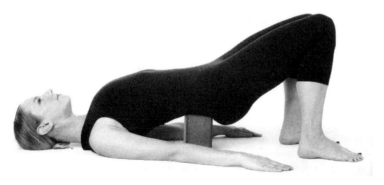

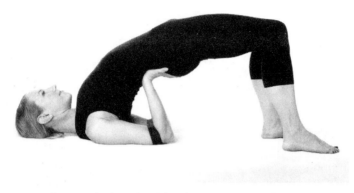

3. Strap your elbows together shoulder distance apart. The strap goes above the elbows. Lift your pelvis and place your hands underneath your lower back.

Ustrasana
Camel Pose

Benefits and How It Works: By arching the entire spine, a partial vacuum is formed between the front parts of the vertebral bodies, which draws the herniated disc material forward, away from the nerve fibers. The global curve also pulls the spinal cord upward through the vertebral canal, enabling it and the nerve roots that project out from it to adjust to regions of compression.

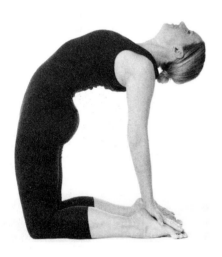

Contraindications: Cervical vertebral displacement, spinal stenosis, severe arthritis, carotid or vertebral arterial disease, late pregnancy, chondromalacia patellae.

The Pose: Kneel with shins together. Point your toes. Take a breath. Reach behind you to place your palms on the soles of your feet. Put weight on the heels as you lift your pelvis and arch your spine. Extend your head back. Make space by opening your hips. Push upward with your heels into the palms of your hands as your pelvis arches forward and your cervical spine arches back. Raise your sternum as high as possible.

LESS CHALLENGING VARIATIONS:

1. Kneel with shins beneath a chair. Toes are pointed. Place your hands on the seat of the chair or your hips. Arch your back against the front of the chair.

2. Kneel and sit back on a large pillow set on the backs of your calves. Grasp your heels and gradually raise your pelvis forward and up, off the pillow.

3. After doing the pose, sit down between your heels, lie back and stretch your arms parallel, palms up, elbows straight, further and further away from your head on the mat. Lower your lumbar spine to the mat (Supta Virasana).

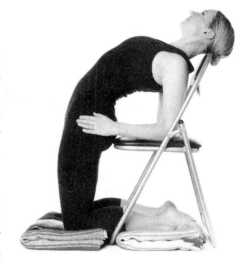

Virabhadrasana I
Warrior I Pose

Benefits and How It Works: Forcibly arches the lumbar and thoracic spine, pulling herniated disc material forward, back underneath the vertebral bodies and out of harm's way.

Contraindications: Severe knee joint derangement, plantar fasciitis, Achilles tendonitis, extreme weakness, concomitant spinal stenosis.

The Pose: Move or jump your legs four and a half feet apart, arms horizontal, palms down. Take two breaths. Turn the left foot 90 degrees to the left and the right foot 30 degrees inward, as you raise your

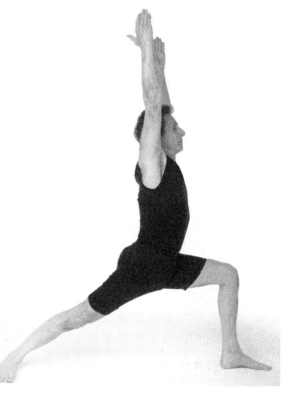

arms to vertical. With your legs straight, swivel your hips so that your navel is facing the same direction as your forward foot. Bend your left knee to a right angle, shin vertical, thigh horizontal. Stretch your fingers and especially your thumbs up to the sky. Breathe evenly for 60 seconds. Return to standing by reversing the sequence.

VARIATIONS:

1. Rest the bent leg's thigh on a chair seat. Place one hand on the bent thigh; use the other for balance by holding the chair back. As you get more secure, work to raise yourself off the chair. Use your leg, not your arms, to do this. Raise your free hand to vertical as balance permits.

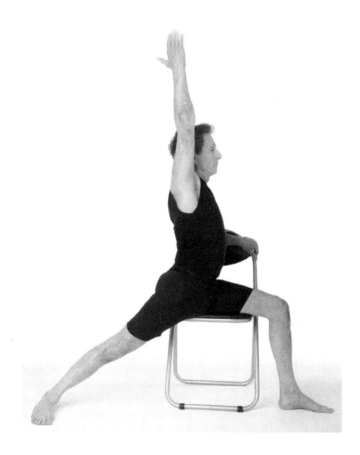

2. Place a block under the forward foot. As you lower your thigh to horizontal, this will further engage the hamstrings and gluteus muscles. This lifts the torso and rocks it backward, reducing the strain of extension of the lower lumbar spine. A wider stance, in which the legs are not in a straight line, eases aligning the torso at right angles to the hips and enhances the therapeutic effects of this pose.

Other Poses for Herniated Disc: Supta Virasana (p. 39), all the Kapotasanas (p. 83), Dhanurasana (p. 194).

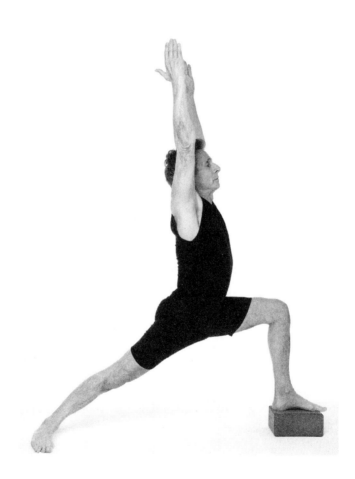

CHAPTER SIX

Stenosis

STENOSIS IS THE narrowing, in one or more places, of the bony canal lead-ing from your brain all the way down to the bottom of your spine. This narrowing can compress the nervous tissue inside the canal. There are three basic causes of this condition, which often affects people as they get older. Arthritis or genetics can, over the course of time, narrow the bony canal in your spine so the nerves just don't have enough room in the smaller space. Second, a bulging or herniated disc or soft tissue may intrude into the central spinal canal and narrow it at that point. The third cause is spondylolisthesis, or slippage of the vertebrae.

Don't get confused: the word "stenosis" means "narrow." Therefore the same word is also used to describe the narrowing of the little neuroforamina—openings through which nerves *exit* the spine—which usually happens with a herniated disc. The central spinal canal leading down from the brain is what we're talking about in this chapter.

You can do some self-diagnosis here. Neuroforaminal stenosis usually gets better when you arch your back and worse when you flex (bend forward). Central spinal stenosis gets better when you flex your spine and worse when you extend it (arch backward).

Narrowing of the bony canal and swelling of the ligamentum flavum, a soft tissue inside the spinal canal, will make the spinal canal narrower. And then, as we age, things that go wrong accumulate. You are more likely to have slippage of one vertebra on another so that they are not exactly aligned. The discs themselves shrink and get thinner and therefore neurological material and the linings all the way up the spine get thicker, like a rubber band that isn't stretched. Even though this involves the whole spinal cord, the pain, numbness and paraesthesias are often only roughly symmetrical; they may not occur, say, in the same toe on both feet, but sometimes they may.

Surgery is sometimes necessary for stenosis. But yoga can help.

Parsvottanasana
Side Stretch Pose

Benefits and How It Works: Gently curves the lumbar spine forward while stretching the hamstrings one leg at a time. This elongates and thereby thins the ligaments inside the spine, creating more room for the nervous tissue there. You can modify the depth of the pose without changing the alignment.

Contraindications: Total hip replacement, herniated disc (any level of the spine), severe osteoarthritis, severe osteoporosis, pregnancy, plantar fasciitis, bicipital tendinitis.

The Pose: Stand with your feet four feet apart. Turn your right foot out 90 degrees, your left foot 30 degrees inward. Inhale as you interlock your fingers behind your back, elbows straight. Pivot 90 degrees, aligning your navel with your right big toe. Take a breath and puff out your chest as you slowly throw your head back. Bend forward from your hips with your neck still extended. Raise your straight arms and hands away from the back of your torso.

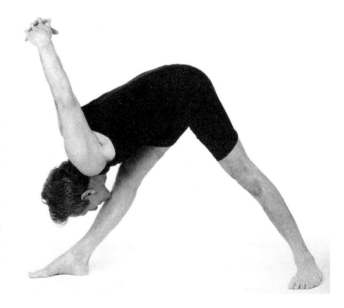

LESS CHALLENGING VARIATION:
If you have trouble balancing in the pose, you can place your hands on a wall or chair in front of you. The goal here is to maintain a relatively straight back.

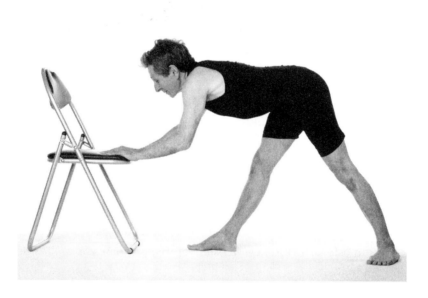

Janusirsasana
Head to Knee Pose

Benefits and How It Works: Similar to Parsvottanasana, this pose gently curves the lumbar spine forward while stretching the hamstrings one leg at a time. In addition, it lengthens the spine, thinning the spinal cord. By "flossing" the spinal cord inside the spinal canal, the pose allows the fibers to rearrange themselves in a less constricted way.

Contraindications: Herniated disc, hamstring tear, osteoporosis, ischial bursitis.

Helpful Hint: If you have difficulty bending from your hips, sit on a folded blanket.

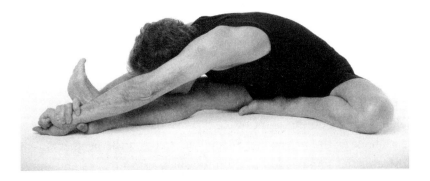

The Pose: Sit on a flat surface with your legs stretched out in front of you. Bend your left knee, pressing the left foot high up on the right thigh. With your back straight, bend your torso forward from your hips. Grasp your left wrist with your right hand at your right foot's arch.

LESS CHALLENGING VARIATION:

If you can't reach your toes, loop a belt around the foot.

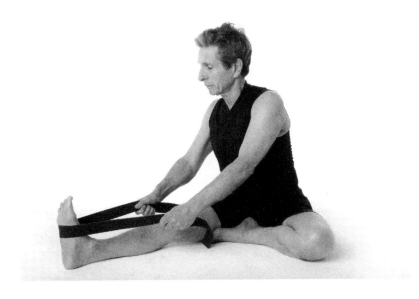

Paschimottanasana
Seated Forward Bend Pose

Benefits and How It Works: This pose helps in two ways. First, by pulling on the sciatic nerve in the legs, the pose slides the spinal cord back and forth a few millimeters within the spinal canal. Mobilizing the spinal cord in this way allows it to seek the point of least resistance, minimizing the pressure brought about by the narrowing. Second, it stretches the ligaments that line the inside of the spinal column, thinning them as a rubber band thins as it stretches, providing more room for the crowded spinal cord.

Contraindications: Vertebral compression or other fracture, -ostomies, ischial bursitis, herniated disc, osteoporosis, severe hip arthritis.

Helpful Hint: If you have difficulty folding from your hips, sit on a folded blanket.

The Pose: Sit on a flat surface with your legs stretched out parallel to each other, inner ankles together. Inhale and lengthen your spine. Bend forward from your hips as you exhale. Grasp your feet, or catch one hand with the other beyond them, or hold a belt looped across the soles of your feet. Keep your ankles close together and dorsiflexed. Reach forward, not down. Rest

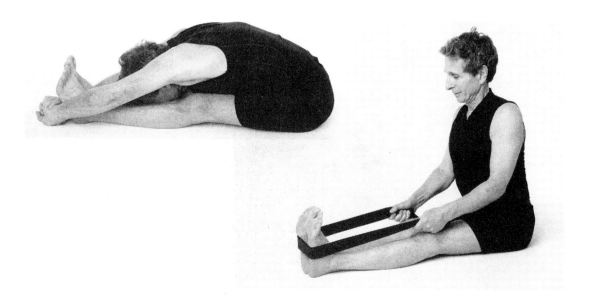

your forehead and cheekbones and, if possible, your chin on the fronts of your legs. Relax your elbows; let the weight of your elbows pull you down. Breathe slowly and evenly to reduce any discomfort.

Floating Dandasana
Floating Staff Pose

Benefits and How It Works: Reduces overarching (lordosis) of the lumbar spine. Strengthens abdominal musculature, favoring relative flexion of the lumbar spine and improving posture while reducing spondylolisthesis.

Contraindications: Carpal tunnel syndrome, wrist, elbow or shoulder instability, extreme hypertension.

The Pose: Sit erect on the floor between two blocks, legs extended in front of you, ankles in contact. Taking a firm grip on the blocks, exhale and raise your torso and pelvis as far off the floor as possible. Raise your straight legs until they are horizontal.

LESS CHALLENGING VARIATION:
Lift one leg at a time.

Other Poses for Central Spinal Stenosis: Krounchasana (p. 224), Ardha Baddha Padma Paschimottanasana (p. 192), Trianga Mukhaikapada Paschimottanasana (p. 223).

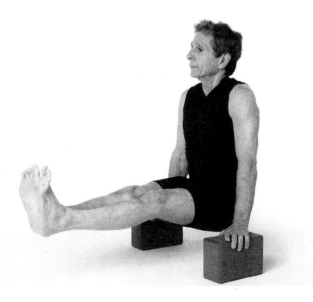

CHAPTER SEVEN

Piriformis Syndrome

THE FIRST TIME I saw piriformis syndrome was in 1986 when I was a young attending physician at Albert Einstein College of Medicine in New York. An orthopedic surgeon came into the room where I was doing EMG (electromyography—tests of nerve conduction). This fellow, whom I knew slightly, had his charge nurse—the head nurse in the operating room—with him. She was in terrific pain and needed an EMG immediately, the surgeon told me. She was a nice thirty-five-year-old woman who had severe bilateral sciatica. MRIs hadn't been invented yet, but the surgeon said the patient's CT scan was normal; she didn't have a herniated disc or spinal stenosis. "I think it may be piriformis syndrome," he said. I had never heard of piriformis syndrome. I said, "There's no EMG test for that." He threw his hands up to the sky and said, "Make one up!" Then he paused briefly and made a suggestion. "Figure out something functional." And he left the room.

At first I thought I would compare one of the nurse's legs with the other, but the condition was bilateral; whatever condition it was, it was probably in both legs. So I decided to compare each leg with itself. She was lying on her stomach on the plinth. While she was lying there in that position I used the EMG to study how well the Achilles tendon reflex worked. Then I moved her leg so that the piriformis muscle was stretched over the sciatic nerve and checked the same reflex. This really hurt, but the result was immediate: the reflex was delayed significantly on both sides. I was surprised and actually happy. Here I was, a young neophyte who knew absolutely nothing about piriformis syndrome and couldn't even remember having heard of it. And now, though I had done a lot of these standard tests for other conditions with my great teacher, Edward F. Delagi, I seemed to have invented a new one. And at the same time I was seeing something totally new. I was giving a patient a diagnosis—her only chance of getting the help she needed.

The surgeon came back to check on his patient and colleague half an hour later. I told him what I had found. He accepted my discovery and diagnosis matter-of-factly, as if he had expected it all along. The next day he operated on her. It was a pretty big deal to me. I scrubbed and brought my camera to take photos of the surgery so the residents could see. Looking into the incisions in the buttock, it was obvious that on both sides the piriformis muscle had compressed the sciatic nerve. The tissue covering these large nerves had markedly thinned just where the muscles were closest to them, and the tiny blood vessels that support the nerve were worn away at the same places.

It was a relatively simple operation because the piriformis muscle lies just below the gluteus maximus, the muscle closest to the surface of the buttock. The nurse was back on duty a week or two later, completely cured.

It was an impressive experience for me, and it piqued my interest in piriformis syndrome. I spent the next seven years as a doctor keeping my eyes open for it. During that time I learned that few people knew about this condition and even fewer in the medical profession believed it existed.[1] It's a little like sacroiliac joint derangement in that way; many physicians and researchers argue that neither exists and the pain attributed to them is caused by other problems.[2] To me, that only made it more fascinating. I believed patients when they said they had that kind of pain, and my test confirmed that some of them did. I found thirty-four cases that I was able to document using the test I invented that placed the leg in flexion, adduction and internal rotation—giving it the acronym of the FAIR test. I wrote up my research and published the article in the *Archives of Physical Medicine and Rehabilitation* seven years after that first case.[3]

Strangely, though I was able to diagnose these patients, many of whom were desperate, and even though I was a specialist in physical medicine and rehabilitation, I didn't know many ways to treat the condition. Often I sent the patients for surgery to the surgeon I had worked with at Albert Einstein. I also prescribed physical therapy, which seemed to help. In the meantime, my little paper caught the eye of the lay press and an article appeared in the *New York Times*.[4]

The morning the article was published, I was inundated with patients who thought they had piriformis syndrome. Since the article was syndicated and appeared in many countries, something wonderful happened. The international therapeutic community, many of whom were more familiar with piriformis syndrome than I was, reached out to me with treatment ideas.

Soon after I began using their suggestions, I realized there were yoga poses that did the same thing and sometimes did it better. Stretching of the piriformis muscle, while it sometimes caused pain, often gave the patient relief soon afterward. I began to think about yoga for this problem, which I believe accounts for a large part of what the medical profession classifies as "lower back pain." In many cases I saw, the piriformis muscle was in spasm that needed to be relieved.

Yoga, I realized, is precise. I could target the piriformis muscle with all sorts of stretches. One pose (Matsyendrasana) would stretch it from the torso, another (Marichyasana) would stretch it from the thigh, below, and Parivrtta Parsvakonasana would elongate it by scissoring the legs together. Sometimes it was almost laughably easy to cure a person on the spot, such as on one occasion a few years ago when I was at a medical convention in Hawaii. A neurologist from Arkansas sitting next to me at a luau told me he had terrible buttock pain that had been going on for ten years and he didn't know what was causing it. We got up from the table and went a little distance from the party. I showed him Parivrtta Trikonasana. Then he had his first painless dinner in a decade. Later he wrote from Little Rock to thank me.

Two years after her first *New York Times* article about my research appeared, science writer Jane Brody did another, and reported that she had never had as much reader response to a column, even those about breast cancer.[5] Again, a flood of hurting patients called my office. As time went on, I discovered that I was not the only person in the medical community researching this problem.[6] In Los Angeles, Dr. Aaron Filler had begun to use a technique called magnetic resonance neurography (MRN) to provide graphic structural evidence of piriformis syndrome. Elsewhere, researchers were discovering that this condition may account for a good deal of sciatica.[7]

What Is Piriformis Syndrome?

The sciatic nerve leaves the pelvis and begins its course down the back of the thigh by crossing just beneath the piriformis muscle. About 15 percent of the time, part or all of the nerve passes through it. In evolutionary terms, the muscle first appears in lizards, and though it is important to their ability to leap and bound, in humankind it is a weak abductor and external rotator of the flexed thigh. One of the chief functions of the piriformis muscle is to cushion and protect the sciatic nerve. However, like the chain guard on a bicycle, the purpose of which is just to prevent complications with the chain, sometimes the piriformis muscle gets into trouble itself. If the muscle gets too tight or is scarred, it can compress the nerve. When that happens it causes sciatica, and in some cases it can damage the sciatic nerve.

The most frequent complaint patients have is pain in the buttock when sitting; pain after exercise is the second most common symptom. Usually there is tenderness toward the middle of the buttock; usually moderate pressure there will bring on the sciatica. Pressure almost invariably hurts.

The best way to diagnose piriformis syndrome without using technical means is to have the patient lie on the unaffected side and bend hips and knees to 90 degrees. Now you can perform three tests: draw a line (an imaginary line will do) from the greater trochanter—the bony part of the thigh that comes closest to the surface of the skin—to the sciatic notch. This is about a 30-degree diagonal going upward and inward toward the body's midline from the trochanter. Press the buttock just about at the midpoint of that line. This is where the sciatic nerve ducks out of the pelvis in close relation to the piriformis muscle, and usually will be tender in people with piriformis syndrome.

Secondly, ask the person to lift the leg (abduct it) in that same position, as you press downward near the knee to gauge its strength. You can check it against the same movement on the other side Usually there is weakness—due to reflex inhibition at the spinal cord level—on the side with piriformis syndrome. This test, devised by Dr. J. B. Pace many years ago, is quite sensitive.

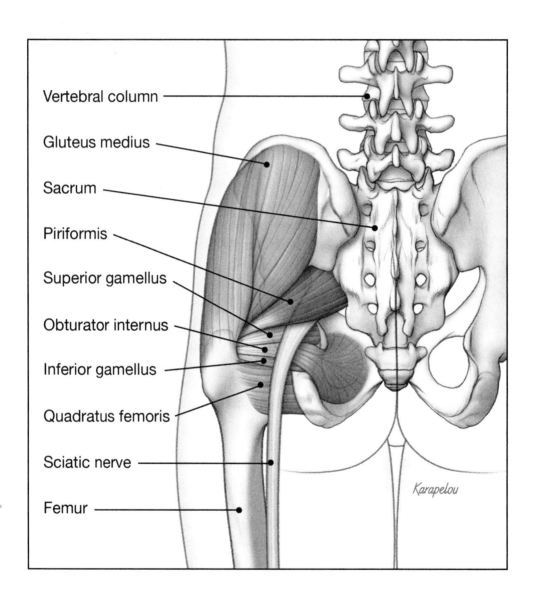

Vertebral column

Gluteus medius

Sacrum

Piriformis

Superior gamellus

Obturator internus

Inferior gamellus

Quadratus femoris

Sciatic nerve

Femur

Karapelou

Third, still in the same position, tell the person to relax the leg and you adduct it, being careful that the patient stays on his or her side and does not just turn over, navel downward, toward you. One way to do this is to press the flexed knee down on a diagonal, toward the patient, not to press straight down. This diagonal pressure on the knee controls the hip quite well. If adduction hurts in the buttock, it's a sign of piriformis syndrome. If it hurts in the groin, that's usually hip arthritis.

Causes of Piriformis Syndrome

Many things can bring on piriformis syndrome. People who sit for hours at a desk—a huge number of us—are at risk. It can be an overuse injury: activities such as hitting too many golf balls at the driving range or running more than three miles a day can send the piriformis muscle into a spasm strong enough to compress the sciatic nerve. The combination of sitting for long periods and doing vigorous physical exercise without much time between these activities can bring on a tightening or clenching of the muscle. So, if you jog in the morning before getting in your car, going to your office and settling in at your desk, make sure you put some time and other activities between your exercise and your sitting. Sitting in a small car while commuting long distances has produced extremely painful piriformis syndrome in many of my patients—so many of them that at one time I could almost guess the make of the car my patient was driving! Mercedes and Hondas were definitely suspect. And then there are those shoes—the sneakers with the round bottoms that are supposed to be good for the wearers. One study showed that people with osteoarthritis of the knee who wore those shoes a lot were prone to piriformis syndrome.[8]

Through trial and error I have seen that stretching the piriformis muscle relieves spasm and stiffness and often helps alleviate pain in the buttock. I have also learned that stretching doesn't work if there is scarring or an anatomical abnormality. In those cases—less than 5 percent of the more than 17,500 I've seen and generally identified through EMG, MRI and MRN—surgery is usually effective. The vast majority of patients, however, benefit greatly from yoga and have need for little else.

Parivrtta Trikonasana
Revolved Triangle Pose

Benefits and How It Works: Since the piriformis muscle abducts the thigh, adducting the thigh will stretch the muscle. Maintaining your whole foot on the floor will balance the muscular forces in the upper leg. Imbalance between adductors and abductors is often why the syndrome arises.

Contraindications: Pregnancy, herniated lumbar disc, acute sacroiliac joint derangement, severe spinal arthritis.

The Pose: Stand with feet three to three and a half feet apart, left foot turned out 90 degrees, right foot turned in 30 degrees, arms stretched out horizontally. Take a breath. Exhale and twist to your left as you bend forward, pivoting your right hip forward until your right hand rests on the floor or a block on the outside of your left foot. Scissor your legs together and lengthen your spine. Draw your shoulderblades together. Your shoulderblades should be in the plane defined by the intersection of your legs. Make your torso narrow and long. Breathe normally for 30 seconds, then repeat on the other side.

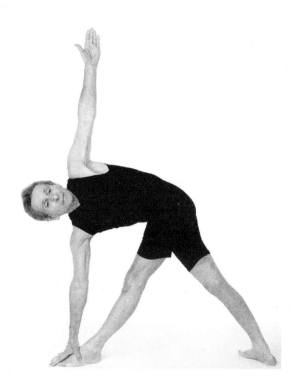

LESS CHALLENGING VARIATIONS:

1. Stand facing a wall with your back foot close to it and your front foot six inches away. Lean against the wall after you twist, getting your back to contact the wall as broadly as possible. If it is difficult to reach the floor, place your hand on a block or a chair. Using the wall and the chair together will help you work on the pose without worrying about your balance.

2. Begin with your back to the wall. Press the forward leg's arm against the wall to twist; use the other arm for balance. This is the least challenging version.

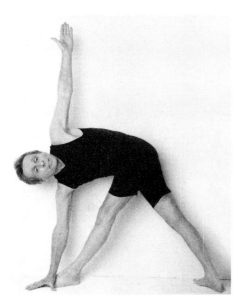 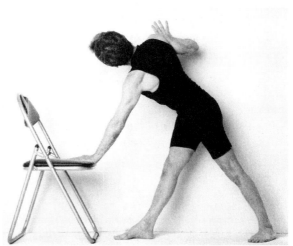

Ardha Matsyendrasana I
Seated Half Twist Pose

Benefits and How It Works: While Parivrtta Trikonasana stretches the piriformis muscle the long way, Matsyendrasana stretches it diagonally. No balance is required; this pose may be used by almost anyone who can sit.

Contraindications: Pregnancy, ischial or trochanteric bursitis, herniated disc, severe kyphosis or scoliosis.

The Pose: Sit tall. Bend your right knee, placing your right heel just to the left of your left hip. The side of your right thigh and calf will rest on the floor. Bend your left knee and place the sole of your left foot on the floor beside your right thigh. The left shin is vertical. Twist your torso to the left, placing the back of your right armpit on the outside of your left knee. Walk your left hand behind yourself, keeping your shoulders even. As you exhale, use the left knee as a fulcrum to gently twist your body further to the left. If possible, catch your right wrist with your left hand. Inflate both the right and left sides of your chest as you gently breathe.

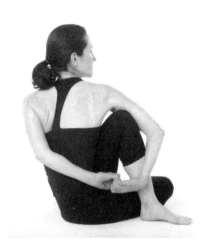

LESS CHALLENGING VARIATIONS:

1. Retain the forward arm straight beside the outside of the vertical shin; walk your other hand as far behind yourself as possible. Remember to keep the back straight and look straight forward.

2. Just grasp your left knee with your right hand and revolve your torso as much as is safe and comfortable.

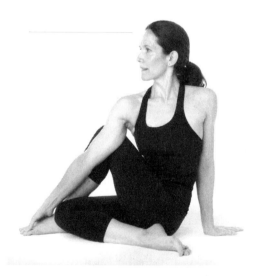

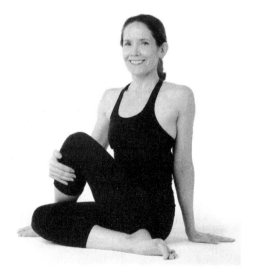

3. Sit about half way back on the seat of a chair so you can feel both feet pressing into the floor. Take hold of the left side of the chair with your right hand. Slide your left arm behind the back of the chair as far as possible and hold on to it there. Soften the abdominal muscles—front, side and back—as you use your arms to twist safely and comfortably.

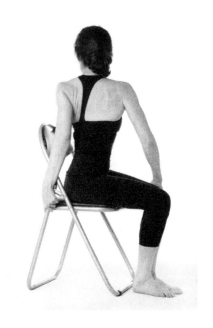

Parivrtta Parsvakonasana
Revolved Side Angle Pose

Benefits and How It Works: Coordinates a stretched piriformis muscle with major muscle groups above and below it. Stretches the piriformis muscle on a unique diagonal.

Contraindications: Poor balance, herniated disc, most types of hernia, severe knee or hip arthritis, anterior cruciate or medial meniscal tear, pregnancy.

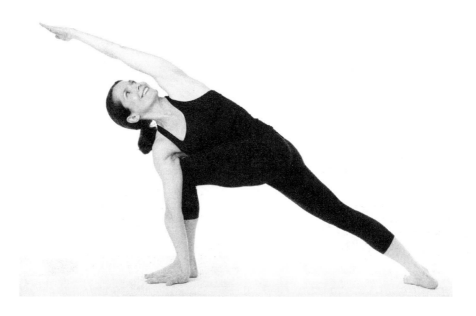

The Pose: Stand with your legs five feet apart, left foot out 90 degrees, right turned 30 degrees inward. Bend the left knee 90 degrees, arms outstretched horizontally. Take two breaths. Thrust your right hip and flank forward to the left, reaching outside your bent knee with your right elbow until the hand is on the floor or on a block, right forearm outside and parallel to the left shin. Extend your left arm diagonally behind your ear and over your head, which is turned upward. Breathe softly and as symmetrically as possible as you extend and lengthen from your right heel to your left fingertips.

LESS CHALLENGING VARIATIONS:

1. Do the pose with your left knee at 90 degrees and right knee on the floor.
2. Use a wall for balance and to improve alignment. Start in a lunge with your right hip and flank against the wall and your left knee bent to 90 degrees, left foot six inches out from the wall. Place your right hand on the floor between the wall and your left foot. Twist your chest to the left, resting your back on the wall. Squeeze your inner thighs toward each other to help you twist. Reach your left arm alongside your left ear. If you have the flexibility, place your right hand on the outside of your left foot.

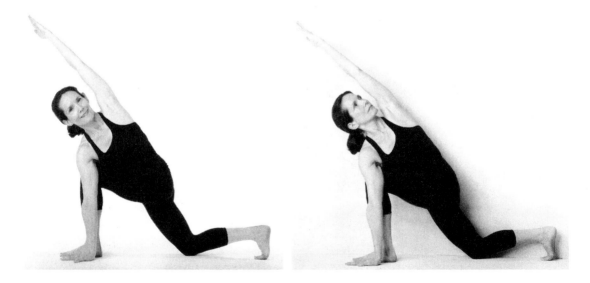

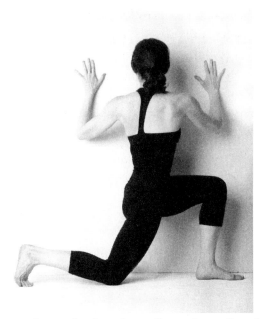

3. Begin the pose with your back to the wall, one knee flexed to 90 degrees, as above, the other leg kneeling. Twist toward the flexed knee. Place both hands on the wall to control and cautiously intensify the twist. Keep your vertebrae in a straight line as you revolve them.

Kapotasana I
Pigeon Pose, Modified

Benefits and How It Works: Stretches the piriformis muscle when the forward leg is flexed more than 90 degrees—the familiar situation while sitting—without aggravating a herniated disc. When the hip is flexed more than 90 degrees, the piriformis muscle slips in front of the femoral bone's round head and becomes an internal rotator. Therefore the external rotation of Kapotasana stretches it by rolling it up over the bone.

Contraindications: Arching the back this way is possibly harmful in spinal stenosis and spondylolisthesis, but usually not in sacroiliac joint derangement.

Helpful Hints: Square your hips to orient the torso so that it is facing straight forward. Relax the abdominal muscles and inhale while arching your back. Elongate your spine; arch as much as possible in the thoracic spine.

The Pose: Kneel on a mat with a cushion or pillow just behind you. Slide your bent right leg (the piriformis leg) forward, the outside of the thigh and calf against the blanket or floor. At this point your left leg will be behind you. Your right shin will be at an angle, with your right foot under your left groin. Settle down into the position by stretching the right leg forward and the left leg back. Lift your left foot by bending your left knee as you arch backward, reaching above your head and back to grasp the foot with the right hand first and then both hands. (Many people can't do this classical pose. Luckily there are modified versions and alternatives).

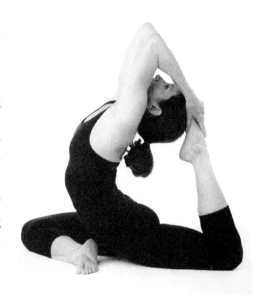

LESS CHALLENGING VARIATIONS:

1. Loop a belt around your left foot at the outset, gradually reaching further back by raising first the left hand to the belt and finally the right hand even closer to the foot. Do this with some speed to generate momentum, enabling you to grab hold of the belt closer to the foot.

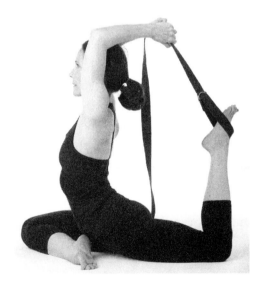

2. Kneel directly in front of a chair. Slide the piriformis leg forward, the outside of the thigh and calf against the floor. Slide the other, straight leg behind you. Holding the front of the seat of the chair, separate your legs further by sliding the piriformis leg forward and the straight leg back. Retain your torso as parallel to the back of the chair as possible as you press against the front of the seat of the chair to comfortably arch your thoracic and lumbar spine, breathing in as you arch, breathing out as you pause in your backward movement.

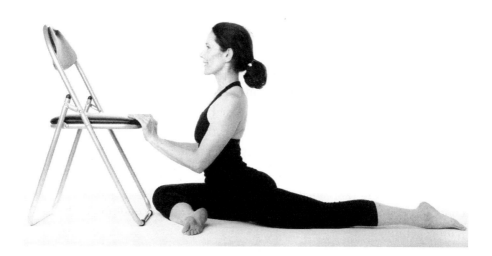

CHAPTER EIGHT

Combination Problems

Now that we have reviewed most of the major sources of back pain and sciatica, we will tackle a problem that arises often: when you have two or more conditions capable of causing back pain and/or sciatica. It can be difficult to accept that you have more than one problem, but this is not a rare occurrence. To make matters worse, the treatments for those conditions may be absolutely opposite. In all cases, and in these cases especially, it is imperative to find out which problem is causing the pain. If more than one condition is active, then the question becomes: which condition is the main pain generator?

Chronic back pain is a problem for millions, and I think a partial explanation is that in many cases more than one condition is responsible. When that happens, an accurate diagnosis is more difficult to achieve for a family doctor and even for a specialist. Worse, chronic pain does more than cause people to lose days of work. It's depressing. It produces anxiety. It makes life so hard that sometimes it doesn't feel worth living. I think it's extremely important to address pain that could be or is becoming chronic and end it as soon as possible. The reasons are obvious. But there is also a less-recognized reason: chronic pain that lasts more than a year seems to have negative effects that last much longer. A study done at Northwestern University shows that a year of chronic back pain actually shrinks the gray matter in the brain by as much as 11 percent, the equivalent of ten to twenty years of normal aging, and that loss is directly related to the duration of the pain.[1] While there is more to be learned, this alone adds to the urgency of relieving back pain not only for the 25 percent of people who report that it is chronic, but for everyone who is at risk for it becoming chronic.

But back to combination problems. There are four types of complex situations that we must identify:

1. *Central spinal stenosis.* Narrowing of the central canal that houses the spinal cord. This may be caused by arthritis, swelling of the linings of the spinal cord or an intervertebral disc that happens to be bulging into the central canal. It can also be caused by spondylolisthesis, where one vertebra has slid forward, backward or to the side of the one below it. The upper vertebrae usually slide forward, and most frequently this occurs at L4–5 or L5–S1. The vertebra may slide more or less out of alignment, depending on your position. And though I am not going to spend a lot of time discussing this condition here, I do want to say that it lowers quality of life drastically for those who have it and that more research is needed to find new methods to relieve it and to put older treatments to better use. Yoga can definitely help.[2]

2. *Neuroforaminal stenosis.* This is the narrowing of the small openings that the nerve roots pass through as they leave the central canal. It can be caused by herniated disc, arthritis and spondylolisthesis.

3. *Piriformis syndrome.* Usually, this is functional—the tightened or spastic piriformis muscle entraps the sciatic nerve as it leaves the pelvis through the buttock. The condition may come and go, but in many cases it comes and stays, sometimes for years.

4. *Sacroiliac joint derangement.* The bones of the sacroiliac joint should fit together perfectly, like the notches of a key fitting into a lock. When the joint is deranged, there is a painful misalignment, often brought about by a misstep or an arduous maneuver (possibly an overly ambitious yoga pose).

These four conditions team up and make people's lives miserable in three common combinations. Finding the main reason for a person's pain is difficult, even with all the available medical technology, which I often use. But I also use my hands-on experience, which people can put to good use at home. When I can't figure out which condition is making my patient hurt, I proceed cautiously and tentatively, trying safe and gentle yoga poses for one condition at a time. I arrive at what helps through careful trial and error. Here are the three most common combination problems I've seen in my practice. It's terrible to see someone suffering from bad back pain and not know how to help, so over the years I've given these situations a lot of thought and have worked hard to find solutions.

Combination Problem 1:
Central Canal Stenosis and Neuroforaminal Stenosis

This is the most common combination of back ailments, in my opinion, and unfortunately it's also the most difficult to deal with. It is complicated by the fact that a third problem, a herniated disc, may be narrowing the neuroforamina and causing the spinal stenosis.

The distinction to focus on here is whether the main problem is in the central canal that contains the nerve fibers that descend and ascend from and to the brain (central canal stenosis), or in the small openings through which the nerve roots exit the central canal on their way to the legs (neuroforaminal stenosis). Yoga that emphasizes flexion and most nonsurgical treatments for central canal stenosis are harmful for the neuroforaminal condition, and yoga treatment for a neuroforaminal narrowing which stresses extension poses is painful for most people who have central canal stenosis. So making up your mind about which condition is the chief cause of the pain is critical.

You can examine yourself to decide which is the main pain generator. Let's first discuss central spinal stenosis.

CENTRAL SPINAL STENOSIS

In central spinal stenosis, the pain, weakness, numbness and paraesthesias may not be exactly symmetrical, but you usually feel them on both sides. For example, the right foot may be numb, and the left calf painful and tingling. The symptoms are often intensified by extension and relieved by flexion. This is the key to more detailed examination: we can actually use yoga to help make the diagnosis of the main pain generator when stenosis is the issue. But proceed gently, and with great caution, and never intentionally try to treat stenosis with yoga twists.

If you have central spinal stenosis, from whatever cause, you'll probably find it worsens with poses like Locust (p. 59), Bridge (p. 60) and Camel (p. 62), and is relieved by forward bends such as Dandasana (p. 31), Janusirsasana (p. 34), Paschimottanasana (p. 70) and Adho Mukha Virasana (p. 25).

NEUROFORAMINAL STENOSIS

Extension helps and flexion exacerbates this condition so much that it is actually capable of worsening a disc herniation. Poses like Locust, Bridge and Camel will relieve pain, and poses with ever so little flexion such as Dandasana, Janusirsasana and Paschimottanasana will be painful and could even cause injury. (These poses are detailed on the pages given above.) So be extremely tentative and go forward little by little, with extreme care. How should you start this process? Since extension will improve disc herniation and will cause pain but will not further injure people with central canal stenosis, it is wisest to start your yogic self-diagnosis with these postures. If you have strong reason to believe that spinal stenosis is causing your pain, then starting with flexion postures might make sense, but since you run the risk of actually increasing the severity of your problem on a long-term basis and enlarging the herniation if one exists, you are generally advised to begin with extension.

You can use further clues to make this important distinction between the two types of narrowing. Central canal stenosis from anything but a herniated disc is more likely to come on very slowly, almost insidiously. Neuroforaminal stenosis often (but not always) stems from a discrete and identifiable event such as heavy lifting, especially with simultaneous twisting, or something traumatic such as an accident or a fall. You might be able to help yourself with a big, arching "Oh what a beautiful morning" kind of stretch.

WHAT TO DO

The pain from neuroforaminal stenosis often grows with mild gentle twists (which you are using just for diagnostic purposes), is worse when twisting to the side of the pathology, and is often temporarily relieved by twists and tilts away from it toward the healthy side. Parivrtta Trikonasana (p. 78) provides excellent trials for twisting; Parighasana (p. 27) is good for tilting. Parivrtta Janusirsasana (p. 45) does a little of both twisting and tilting.

WHEN IN DOUBT

If you cannot confidently determine whether it is central canal stenosis or a neuroforaminal narrowing that is causing your pain, you should begin by doing some cautious, mild yoga, starting with the poses for the condition that seems more likely. Go slowly. If nothing changes after a few days, go slightly forward on your chosen path. Continue until your trial seems to be working or is consistently causing more pain. If you are improving, you should confidently but gradually increase the chosen program. If the course you're on is pretty certainly increasing your pain, then stop it and begin working with the other hypothesis, paying close attention to how you feel. If you were trying flexion postures for possible central spinal stenosis, then try extension postures for neuroforaminal stenosis. Within ten days you should have a good idea of which condition you have to contend with.

WHEN ALL ELSE FAILS

What if trying yoga to treat both conditions does not work, or seems to be making you worse? In that case, see a physiatrist or sports medicine physician and do not settle for anything less than a diagnosis. Insist on tests, and if you cannot get a definite diagnosis, see another doctor. It is challenging to identify the pain-causing culprit in this situation, even for the sophisticated contemporary specialist, since an MRI and conventional EMG will show both conditions but will not give much of a clue about which one should be treated first. I have written a book—*Functional Electromyography: Provocative Maneuvers in Electrodiagnosis* (Springer, Science and Business Media, 2011)—about novel electrodiagnostic methods that can make this distinction, but the techniques are not widely used at this writing.

Combination Problem 2:
Piriformis Syndrome and Neuroforaminal Stenosis or Central Canal Stenosis Caused by Herniated Disc

You may have sciatica caused by (and confirmed with a diagnosis of) piriformis syndrome. In addition, you may have a herniated disc causing central canal stenosis or neuroforaminal stenosis. Unfortunately, the twisting poses that are so helpful for piriformis syndrome are positively harmful for herniated disc. As I've already emphasized, enthusiastic or powerful twisting is dangerous for anyone who has spinal stenosis, herniated disc, or spondylolisthesis from whatever cause. Here is another example of the importance of determining the operant diagnosis—which condition is causing more than half the pain.

The distinction we must make in this case is whether the source of the pain is in the spine or in the buttock. Since the tests for the conditions in the spine will not injure the piriformis muscle, but the tests for piriformis syndrome may do further harm in the spine, it is best to begin testing for the spinal conditions.

SPINAL CONDITIONS

Both spinal stenosis and spondylolisthesis usually become more symptomatic when you arch your back, and if you haven't been reading above, remember to be careful of all twists. Poses like Salabhasana (p. 59), Setu Bandhasana (p. 60) and Ustrasana (p. 62) may increase the pain. Herniated discs become more painful with flexion or bending forward. Therefore pain may mount with Dandasana (p. 31), Janusirsasana (p. 34) and Paschimottanasana (p. 70). Remember, the poses that increase pain in herniated disc will likely relieve pain due to central spinal stenosis, and vice versa. None of these will do much to help or hurt with piriformis syndrome.

WHAT TO DO

The pain from a herniated disc often grows worse when you do gentle twists and tilts to the side of the herniation. On the other side of the coin, one can often temporarily relieve that pain with twists and tilts away from the site of the damage to the disc. Matsyendrasana (p. 42) and Parivrtta Trikonasana (p. 78) provide excellent trials for twisting, Parighasana (p. 27) is good for tilting, and Parivrtta Janusirsasana (p. 45) does both.

If testing yourself this way is strongly persuasive, then proceed to the postures given in chapter 5, "Herniated Disc," and chapter 6, "Stenosis." Those poses won't harm people who also have piriformis syndrome. In fact, the conditions you are treating frequently exacerbate and occasionally even *cause* piriformis syndrome, so treating them may help minimize the piriformis complaints as well.

PIRIFORMIS SYNDROME

We do not always need yoga to help with a diagnosis of piriformis syndrome. The pain usually worsens with sitting, and usually there is a spot near the middle of the buttock that is tender to a moderate push. Please note the word "usually" here. There are times when you should see a physician, because these simple tests, while reliable, are not perfect. In this syndrome, pain is usually relieved *after* twists such as Parivrtta Trikonasana (p. 78), Marichyasana I (p. 41), Matsyendrasana (p. 42) and Parivrtta Parsvakonasana (p. 81). The poses themselves may be uncomfortable, particularly at first, but careful and gentle, gradually progressive practice will generally alleviate or end the pain and other uncomfortable symptoms of piriformis syndrome.

WHAT TO DO

If, after testing, it appears that piriformis syndrome is likely to be causing the most pain, you still must take particular care. The twisting used to relieve piriformis syndrome will be harmful to people with herniated discs, stenosis or spondylolisthesis, even if those conditions are not actively causing the pain when you start. Unfortunately, these conditions often coexist in latent, almost painless form with piriformis syndrome. If you have both piriformis syndrome and one or more of the other diagnoses, you should start simply.

A Version of Anantasana
Ankle Under Couch Pose

This pose can be useful if you have piriformis syndrome coupled with spinal issues. Although it is a far cry from the classic Anantasana (Side Reclining Leg Lift), that is its closest relative in the yoga family. It takes advantage of the agonist–antagonist reflex so useful in yoga.

Note: In severe cases it is best to start with this pose rather than the somewhat more challenging and perilous Parivrtta Ardha Chandrasana. If you can do more than this, try the next pose.

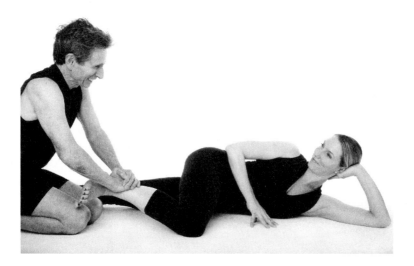

Benefits and How It Works: Uses isometric adduction and internal rotation to activate the agonist–antagonist reflex. It will relax the piriformis muscle, an abductor and external rotator, without negatively affecting the spine.

Contraindications: Total hip replacement, knee replacement, trochanteric bursitis (on the opposite side).

The Pose: Lie on the side that doesn't hurt, with the involved hip and knee bent to 80–90 degrees. Have a friend hold your top ankle down, or hook your ankle under a sturdy object such as a couch or heavy chair. Press your knee down into the floor as you raise your ankle upward into your friend's hand or against the underside of the furniture.

Parivrtta Ardha Chandrasana
Revolved Half Moon Pose

Benefits and How It Works: The pelvis twists on the thigh, stretching the piriformis muscle, but the torso rotates with the pelvis, minimizing torque that might negatively affect neuroforaminal stenosis, spondylolisthesis or central spinal stenosis.

Contraindications: Total hip prosthesis, rotator cuff syndrome, carpal tunnel syndrome, pregnancy.

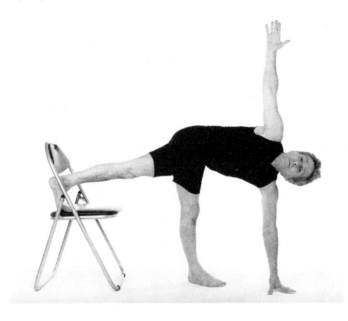

Helpful Hints: Rest the horizontal leg on a chair behind you for stability and to help you twist more. When you're ready to lift your horizontal leg off the chair, you will have achieved a modicum of control over the piriformis muscle. This is a difficult pose and balance is a real issue. At first you may need to stabilize your left leg against a wall, or on a chair that is against a wall.

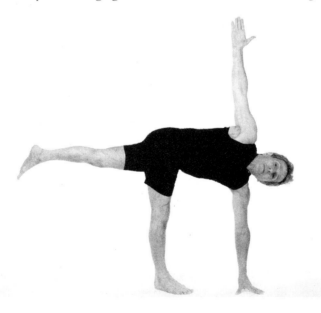

You can also start out with a second chair facing away from you, placed a little in front of your supporting leg. Basically you will be horizontal, suspended and twisted on one leg, with one chair by the feet and another toward the shoulders, with one hand on it. So if your left foot and right hand are down on the floor, and your right leg is stretched out horizontally, your left hand will be on the other chair. To minimize the possibilities of falling and overtwisting, please read the entire pose with the notes and be sure you understand them before attempting it.

The Pose: Stand with feet three to three and a half feet apart. Turn the right foot out 90 degrees and the left foot inward 30 degrees. Bend your right knee moderately as you pivot your left hip forward, resting your left hand on the floor 9–12 inches in front of your right foot. Get secure in that position before raising your left leg to horizontal and turning your entire torso toward your right thigh. As you do this lift your right arm to vertical, and lengthen, thrusting your left heel backward and your head forward. Breathe freely. Stretch from head to toe.

WHEN TESTS FOR PIRFORMIS, STENOSIS, SPONDYLOLISTHESIS FAIL

Here again you may find that all the tests are negative, or all the tests are positive, or for one reason or another you're still confused about what to do. Of course you want to avoid doing anything that might be dangerous. Let's say you've started with the tests for spinal problems and have not had decisive results. Then you've tried to confirm that piriformis syndrome is the active condition, and again have come up with no firm conclusion. Your first option is to proceed to do yoga for the most likely spinal condition, knowing that treatment will not make the piriformis syndrome worse. Seeing how that goes, you may happily find that you're on the right road. If not, then I advise seeing a physiatrist or sports physician. As it happens, my book *Functional Electromyography: Provocative Maneuvers in Electrodiagnosis* contains an electrophysiological decision procedure for central spinal stenosis vs. neuroforaminal stenosis, and provides a reasonably definitive answer to the question: "Do I have piriformis syndrome?"

Combination Problem 3:
Sacroiliac Joint Derangement and Piriformis Syndrome

Many people agree with me that sacroiliac joint derangement is one cause of piriformis syndrome. Some even suggest that a tight piriformis muscle can cause sacroiliac joint derangement, which I doubt because I don't think the muscle is strong enough to disrupt the joint. I believe the piriformis muscle is of interest not because of its strength, but because of its position just above the sciatic nerve. But the problem with the dual diagnosis is the same one we have already encountered twice before: the treatment for piriformis syndrome may aggravate sacroiliac derangement. Here, though, the distinction between the two problems may be more difficult to make.

DISTINGUISHING BETWEEN SACROILIAC JOINT DERANGEMENT AND PIRIFORMIS SYNDROME

Sacroiliac joint derangement feels worst while getting up from sitting, getting out of the back seat of a car, or possibly when leaning forward to do something like brush your teeth, lift a suitcase or wash the dishes. Piriformis syndrome is most painful when you are actually sitting.

While piriformis syndrome may (though it doesn't always) produce radiating symptoms and sciatica, the pain of sacroiliac joint derangement is almost invariably located just where the joint is, an inch or two off the midline of your body and along the bony interface of the iliac bone and the sacrum: that is, below your waist and above your buttocks. It never causes numbness, paraesthesias or sciatica. Mild pressure near the middle of the very lower back at that place often brings on the pain. This pain does not go down the leg.

Frequently the pain of sacroiliac joint derangement will shift from side to side. This is because the sacrum is a single, midline bone, and if one side is out of kilter, the angles also have got to be disturbed on the other side. But 90 percent of the time piriformis syndrome occurs only on one side.

You'll need a friend to perform this simple test for distinguishing piriformis syndrome from sacroiliac joint derangement. Let's say you have pain in the right buttock. Lie on your left side and bend both your knees and your hips 90 degrees. Your hips are parallel and your right leg is on top of your left leg. Have your friend hold down the right leg by pressing down on the outside of the right knee. Then attempt to raise your right thigh up, to lift it off the left thigh; your friend's hand is opposing your effort to raise the right thigh. Then turn on your right side and do the same thing with your left leg. If you find that the muscles lifting one thigh are much weaker than those on the other side, it suggests piriformis syndrome. Pain at the sacroiliac joint during this maneuver implicates the sacroiliac joint.

None of the manipulative tests for sacroiliac joint derangement are particularly accurate. This is partially because so many different things can go wrong with this huge, bilateral, saddle-shaped joint, and partially because there is no high-tech way to corroborate them. MRI and X-rays are almost useless, showing little or nothing except in egregious cases such as fracture or infection. In fact, some doctors are reluctant to believe the sacroiliac joint can become deranged! The test that I find the most accurate is the Swedish test known as Gaenslen's sign, which involves lying on a table or chair, lifting one knee toward the chest and allowing the other leg to descend slowly off the side of the table or chair, bringing the weight of it toward the floor. Pain will occur in the sacroiliac joint if SI derangement is the diagnosis.

Note: Although the neurological correspondence between, e.g., pain at the lateral calf and an L5–S1 nerve problem is almost unerringly present, Gaenslen's sign is only 60–70 percent accurate.

WHEN TESTS FAIL

Here again you must weigh the relative strengths of the signs and symptoms to decide where to begin. If nothing pops out at you but you're pretty sure both conditions are present, I recommend starting with the sacroiliac joint poses, since sacroiliac joint derangement may be causing the piriformis pain. Three to four weeks later, the SI joint should be better, but if there is still tenderness in the buttock and pain when sitting, do the poses for piriformis syndrome. Unfortunately, that may aggravate the sacroiliac joint a bit, and in another few weeks you may have to switch back to the yoga for sacroiliac joint pain. But by then you'll likely have engaged the piriformis muscle and improved dynamics in the muscles surrounding the sacroiliac joint, and the job will be far enough along so it will be quite easily tolerable. You can find more information in my books *Yoga for Back Pain, Sciatica Solutions* and *Back Pain.*

IF YOU HAVE HAD AN OPERATION

There is one further complication that is common enough to deserve comment. A number of people have had surgery, successful or not, on their lower backs, and yet afterward have reason to believe they have piriformis syndrome. The syndrome may have developed later, or it may have been the cause of the sciatica for which the surgery was mistakenly performed. In any case, these postsurgical cases are at risk of injury from the twisting poses that are so effective for piriformis syndrome. The version of Anantasana given above is safe. Most of the other poses can be made safe by wearing a lumbosacral corset with posterior steels during the yoga treatment. Just put it on before doing yoga for piriformis syndrome, and take it off afterward. There is no need to wear it at other times, unless it helps.

PART 4

Injuries and Systemic Problems

CHAPTER NINE

Rotator Cuff

THE FIRST TIME I tore my rotator cuff we were in the woods of upstate New York one January for what was supposed to be a fun vacation weekend with our kids and several other families from their school. The main activity was cross-country skiing, because we could all do it and it was so safe—you just couldn't get hurt. Or so I thought. The snow was perfect, and a group of us set out on well-marked trails. There were almost no hills, just small inclines appropriate for inexperienced skiers like the children. But I noticed an icy patch where one of the kids and a parent slid and fell. Nothing serious. I didn't think twice as I skied down that short slope, but it was very slippery and I fell at the bottom. I got up immediately, certain that absolutely nothing was wrong. I felt no pain. But a few seconds later, I realized that I could not lift my right arm.

One of the adults in the party was a neurosurgeon. He used a safety pin to see if I could feel the pinprick. I passed a couple of simple tests. "You're okay," he said. Then another parent, a lawyer, asked me if anything like this had ever happened to me before; was it just the trail that had made me slip? I said I thought it was, and he replied, only partially in jest, "That may be actionable." We both laughed. My wife was watching all this, and because I was smiling and joking she didn't take it seriously, until the neurosurgeon's wife, a nurse, advised that we go home and call an orthopedist. I had an MRI the next morning. It showed a significant but not massive full-thickness rotator cuff tear. Shortly after that, I had surgery.

The pain of the operation was extreme. I lay in my hospital bed, pressing that morphine button as if I were a rat in a test cage. It seemed like only a few hours before a physician friend of mine stopped by to see how I was doing and pronounced me ready for physical therapy. I couldn't believe that PT would help the kind of extreme postsurgical pain that I was feeling but, more or less humoring him, I agreed to try it. A little apple-faced girl who had probably treated a total of two patients in her life moved my arm passively, and within about five minutes my pain had lessened greatly. I asked the nurse to take out the IV; I didn't need the morphine anymore.

I got out of the hospital still quite disabled, having to use my left hand to raise my right arm when I saw patients. I was inundated with patients because of a newspaper article about me that had come out while I was in the hospital, so I embarked on a rehab program in my own facility, where I had my own physical therapists. We all watched my progress carefully. It took three months for me to regain full function and movement of my shoulder with the standard physical therapy methods: six weeks of passive range-of-motion help, six weeks of active assisted range-of-motion exercises and six weeks of active range-of-motion for strengthening after the twelve weeks of inactivity. My own case illustrated what I had read in medical school and elsewhere: that it takes three months to correct a rotator cuff tear whether or not there has been a surgery.

That thinking is changing, however. A recent prizewinning study done at New York City's Hospital for Special Surgery suggests that changes in rehabilitation after rotator cuff surgery might be beneficial.[1] Instead of beginning with passive range of motion, the researchers hypothesize that six weeks of immobilization might work better in the long run because that would reduce production of scar tissue, which is weaker than normal tissue. But more research is needed. And, even if those scientists are correct, I would rather avoid surgery and six weeks of immobilization if I possibly could.

At this point I have no pain in that shoulder and I have complete range of motion. But that isn't true of everyone who has surgery. Some people end up pain-free but without their former range of motion.[2] Others have considerable pain.

About ten years after I had the rotator cuff surgery, I was driving down Seventh Avenue in Greenwich Village with my family when a taxicab cut me off. I jerked the wheel as hard as I could to avoid a crash. I was taking an antibiotic at the time, one that is known to weaken tendons. That sudden, hard pull of the wheel was enough to snap something in my rotator cuff. Here I go again, I thought. This time the tear was on the left side, and this time it was massive. Though it wasn't at all painful, I couldn't raise my arm beyond about 50 degrees. Again I got an MRI. The same surgeon who had operated on my right shoulder took one look and said, "This one is beyond me. It's a massive tear. You'll have to go to one of the great experts." I asked him whether I should do my regular yoga practice, which I've been doing every day my whole adult life. He cautioned me against doing anything that involved the shoulder, and specifically to avoid doing headstand. So I called two of the greatest shoulder experts in New York, and even though I'm a fellow doctor, I couldn't get in to see either one for a month.

One morning about a week later, I still couldn't raise my arm to save my soul. I missed being able to stand on my head, and during my morning practice I decided to do it for a short time, as cautiously as I could. There wasn't any problem getting down on all fours, assuming the correct position and lifting my legs into the air. I stood on my head for a minute or two. Observing the classical Iyengar method, I lifted my shoulders far from the ears, sharing my weight between the cervical spine and the forearms. This felt good. There was no pain. I usually did headstand for half an hour, and that day it was unclear to me how long I could safely stay in the pose.

While I was up there my wife came into the room and said, "Loren, what are you doing? Don't hurt yourself!" I came right down, feeling sheepish. I was about to say that I'd been a little irresponsible when I realized I could raise my arm, vertically and to the side. Both flexion and abduction were absolutely normal and painless. It was strange. It was weird. Though I was happy, I couldn't understand it. I kept trying it and my arm kept working! But I knew I had not healed a massive tear in a couple of minutes.

I took my yoga shorts to work with me that day. When I was there I recruited one of the physical therapists to do an EMG on me while I was standing on my head to test how well my shoulder's nerves and muscles were functioning. We discovered that the subscapularis muscle was active when I stood on my head the Iyengar way, where the shoulders are raised up from the floor quite forcibly. That was pretty surprising, and I wanted to see if it were really true. So I tested myself again while I was abducting that arm—lifting it out to the side—which I couldn't do before standing on my head. The subscapularis was quite active in this position as well.

Since then I've tested it many times with the same results. I've used an eight-channel EMG and taught myself to stand on my head without moving at all for long enough—almost half an hour—to do an MRI. I had a complex CT scan and did many other studies, not only on myself but on my patients. The headstand seemed to work for them too. In my judgment, I have now proven that headstand, which I have modified a little over time, teaches the subscapularis to take over for the injured supraspinatus in the rotator cuff. But it works only if after the headstand the subject stands up straight and immediately abducts and flexes the arm—lifts it to vertical, both out to the side and in front. If the patient raises her arm straight up to the ceiling right after the headstand, she is often "cured" on the spot. That's because the subscapularis works like a kind of cantilever, pulling down the head of the humerus while the deltoid holds the bone in place, and that raises the shaft.

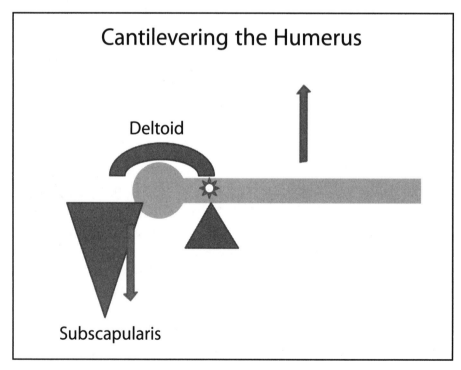

Cantilevering the Humerus

Deltoid

Subscapularis

Under normal conditions, the deltoid lifts the arm from your side to about 80 degrees. At that point its fibers are pulling nearly horizontally and cannot raise the arm further. That's when the supraspinatus comes in and pulls it another 20–30 degrees skyward. After that aid the deltoid has a vertical component to its angle and can do the rest of the job of raising the arm over your head. But in rotator cuff tear, the supraspinatus may be partially torn or actually ripped into two fragments. In that case, abduction or flexion beyond 80 degrees is either very painful or impossible—impossible, that is, unless you can recruit the subscapularis.

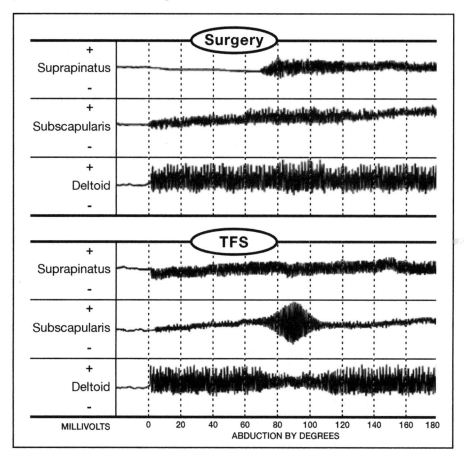

Headstand and some similar maneuvers we will discuss here activate the subscapularis. What takes place afterward occurs because the subscapularis remains active and is easily incorporated into your movements. When you raise your arm to 80 degrees immediately after doing headstand, the deltoid holds the shaft of the bone, gripping it quite close to the shoulder, while the subscapularis pulls downward, and like a cantilever bridge or a seesaw, the long shaft of the humerus rises. After you practice this a few times, the learning becomes permanent. Since using the supraspinatus is painful or useless, it becomes a case of operant conditioning: you are rewarded for using the subscapularis by having your arm rise painlessly, and painfully punished for trying (unsuccessfully) to raise your arm with the supraspinatus. In a short time, the subscapularis becomes your muscle of choice for abduction and flexion.

I've followed patients for twelve years after they've done this maneuver, and even then the subscapularis is still doing its job. In most cases, the supraspinatus does not heal. As far as I can tell, no harm is done because the supraspinatus isn't working. But I suppose that much later it could be a cause of arthritis, which I have also discovered in some patients after ten years. The few cases in which I have confirmed subsequent healing with an MRI have one thing in common: these patients learned the yoga maneuver within the first few weeks of acquiring rotator cuff syndrome. But almost everyone improves.

WHAT IS ROTATOR CUFF TEAR?

The rotator cuff is a group of four muscles that give the shoulder joint stability because their tendons attach to the humerus (the upper arm bone) in such a way as to form a cuff around it. This muscle group also provides force for the arm to rotate inward and outward, abduct, flex and push downward. The muscle that is critical for lifting the arm, the supraspinatus, is small and poorly suited for the task of raising this comparatively long limb, especially at an angle of around 90 degrees, and especially because way out at the end of the arm is a hand that may be holding or swinging something heavy.

This muscle appears in four-legged animals, but it never has the task of working against gravity in a horizontal position for them, and there is never something heavy held in a paw at such a mechanical disadvantage. Perhaps evolution has not caught up with the erect creatures we have become. That's at least a partial explanation of why, when a shoulder injury occurs in a human, it is most often in the supraspinatus tendon, according to the American Academy of Orthopaedic Surgeons.[3]

Experts agree that the major causes of rotator cuff tear, which affects

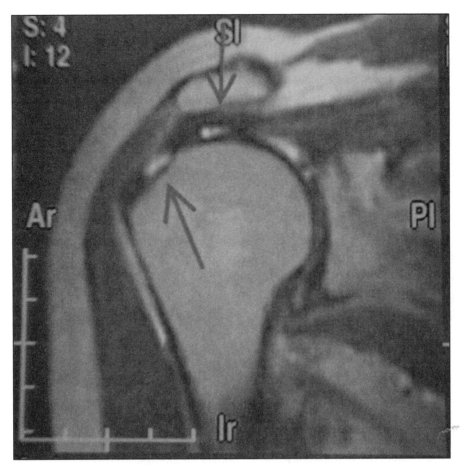

MRI of a supraspinatus muscle torn completely in two.

millions of Americans every year, are repetitive use problems from sports such as tennis, volleyball, baseball, and golf, and tasks that require heavy lifting near 90 degrees. An accident can also cause a rotator cuff tear. Athletes and older people are most prone to have a rotator cuff tear. Sometimes rotator cuff injuries are not symptomatic, and the person who has one may not know it. The research shows that even when there are no symptoms, tears will get bigger during a five-year period for 40 percent of these patients, and 80 percent will develop symptoms sometime down the road after the initial injury.[4] There is some evidence that women with rotator cuff pathology suffer from higher levels of pre- and postoperative disability than men.[5]

An MRI of the shoulder is the best way for a doctor to diagnose a full-thickness rotator cuff tear. Short of that, there are three physical tests that sharply raise suspicion of a tear: the painful arc, the drop arm sign and weakness in external rotation. The first test, the painful arc, simply notes whether it is painful to abduct the arm (bring it out to the side) or to flex the arm (bring it out and raise it in front of you). In each case, you lift the arm until it is over your head. Generally rotator cuff tears start to hurt at about 80 degrees, and if yours does, the test is positive. The drop arm test is done by lowering the arm from overhead, generally with the palm facing downward. In the same two positions, lowering the arm in front of you and on the side, perpendicular to and in the same plane as your torso, respectively, you feel pain at about 90 degrees. Weakness in external rotation is another sign. To test this, hold your arm out horizontally in front of you with elbow bent, and bring your forearm arm up in a windshield wiper motion against mild resistance (which you can apply with the other hand). Pain indicates a rotator cuff tear. If you find that two of these three tests are positive, you probably have a rotator cuff tear.

There are two other considerations. An individual who has had a rotator cuff tear for a while may develop adhesive capsulitis, or frozen shoulder. Whether or not you have pain, frozen shoulder will limit your range of motion, reducing how far you can lift your arm in either direction. These limitations may restrict how much the TFS maneuver (detailed below) can help you, and in extreme cases may prohibit the maneuver altogether.

Secondly, look for any weakness, numbness or paraesthesia in that arm. Neurological problems such as a pinched cervical nerve or entrapment of a nerve are the second most frequent cause of shoulder disability. Systemic conditions such as diabetes are possible culprits too.

Researching My Yoga-Like Method

Many patients came to me for rotator cuff tears before I was sure that this maneuver, which I call the Triangular Forearm Support (TFS), could work immediately to cure pain and restore range of motion. To confirm my results, I sent these patients for one or two physical therapy sessions right after they did the maneuver and raised their arms, and I started keeping track of those

I treated with the TFS, which a superb and resourceful physical therapist named Tova Ovadia helped me modify. The TFS is a headstand or inversion based on the pose of my teacher, B. K. S. Iyengar. You can stand on your head to accomplish it, but you do not have to be able to do that. Those who don't know how to stand on their heads or cannot for various reasons can achieve the same results in other ways described below. One comes directly from Tova.

When I tried to publish a paper detailing my findings, I ran into a lot of difficulty. One editor wrote back saying this was too radical, more or less in the tone of, "Are you kidding?" An orthopedic surgeon at Columbia University Medical School, where I teach, wanted me to dissociate myself from the university because, he said, "This notion is dangerous."

No one wanted to publish it, though by the time I was ready to make my results public I had had success with more than 600 patients. Finally I submitted it to the journal of the International Association of Yoga Therapists (IAYT). They rejected it too. Then, almost incredibly, one of the reviewers had a student with a rotator cuff tear. He tried my method and it worked. A few weeks later they accepted the paper. I don't think that article would ever have been published otherwise.

The first two times I spoke to colleagues about this, they were polite but their attitude was one of barely disguised disbelief. The first time I gave the paper was at the annual meeting of the Association of Academic Physiatrists in Albuquerque in 2004. When I had finished delivering my speech, there was not a sound in the large audience. Not one person applauded. That was when I knew I was onto something. I didn't want to be regarded as a member of the lunatic fringe, but on the other hand, I felt pretty sure that the TFS worked.

In spite of much resistance on the part of conference organizers, I presented my research again in 2005, at the Columbia University Symposium on Alternative Medicine for Pain. I remember well my friend and colleague James Dillard expressing his skepticism. My wife remembers hearing tittering in the audience.

Things changed in the next six years, maybe because word began to get around. At the next International Association of Yoga Therapists conference, I brought a woman up out of an audience of about 350 people. This woman hadn't been able to raise her arm in seven years. With my help she did the TFS. Then she painlessly lifted her arm to the side and straight in front of her to 170 degrees and cured her rotator cuff while on stage. The whole thing, exam and all, took less than ten minutes. She was very excited about being able to lift her arm for the first time in years and she broke into a huge grin, went back to her seat and gleefully lifted that arm over and over again as she listened to the rest of the program.

In 2011 I published another rotator cuff paper in the peer-reviewed journal *Topics in Geriatric Rehabilitation*.[6] That winter I went to Haridwar, India, and spoke to a huge audience (it was also broadcast on cable television to a reported audience of 50 million!) in a room the size of an airplane hangar. The occasion was the First International Symposium on Yoga for Health and Social Transformation. Along with several other physicians and scientists from around the world, I presented my findings to a panel of judges whose mission was to bring scientific investigation to yoga. When I finished, one of them said, "If I ever have a problem with my rotator cuff, I know whom to see." The other presenters were impressive, and I felt they had done more and better work than I had. But after I returned to New York I learned I had been awarded a prize. Still, few clinicians use this method.

It was at that same conference that I unexpectedly and joyfully ran into my teacher, B. K. S. Iyengar, whose headstand had inspired me to do the research. During a briefly held but long remembered conversation he smiled at me and said "You do not own your body; you only rent it."

I've now used the maneuver to help more than 1,200 people with rotator cuff tears and a few other shoulder conditions. It has worked in about 90 percent of cases—nearly 1,100 of the patients I've treated with the TFS. I've followed patients for up to fourteen years, some with several repeats of their MRIs. The maneuver keeps working, enabling people to raise their arms completely, with full strength and without any pain. However, there is slightly more arthritis in the joint as compared with the normal aging process, and the torn tendon does not usually heal. That doesn't matter much, though, since these people have full and unaltered function and no other problems whatever.

Surgery, though expensive and painful, is a frequent solution for those vwith a rotator cuff tear, as it was for me the first time I injured myself. I think anyone with a torn rotator cuff would do well to try the TFS before deciding to have an operation. With surgery or without it, patients who have not done TFS need three months of rehabilitation before full and (hopefully) painless function of the shoulder is restored. The rehab is arduous and it takes a long time to achieve a full cure—if it's achieved at all. That's why patients with whom I have done the TFS maneuver are so grateful. It usually takes only a few minutes and one office visit and, according to my clinical trial, it's effective at least 90 percent of the time.

Almost anyone who has an MRI showing a rotator cuff tear and who has symptoms can benefit from the TFS. It's not necessary to be able to stand on your head. In a few isolated cases, patients have not been able to learn the maneuver. This has sometimes happened with musicians who have been taught to hold a violin, cello or guitar or artists who hold a paintbrush in such a way that their shoulderblades have been overtrained in these activities and strenuously resist being taught a new shoulder dynamic.

WHAT TFS CAN HELP
The TFS maneuver doesn't cure every type of shoulder pain. It worked first on my own massive rotator cuff tear. Although I haven't done blinded clinical trials yet, it seems to be almost as useful for a couple of other problems. It can help with inflammation of the supraspinatus tendon (tendinitis) and with some cases of impingement syndrome, in which the tendon gets compressed between the humerus and the shoulderblade at the top of the shoulder. Impingement syndrome usually causes pain, weakness and loss of range of shoulder motion. Sleeping on the affected shoulder can worsen this condition. The TFS maneuver pulls the head of the arm bone away from the impinging part of the shoulderblade, the acromion, and often relieves it. The TFS can also provide relief from labral tear, which is an injury to the thick "washer" around the shoulder socket. This may be damaged by a specific trauma or worn away in aging. Its symptoms include ache, "catching" of the shoulder with movement and pain that occurs with specific movements. The maneuver has also been sometimes successful with arthritis that involves the top part of the humerus and the glenoid fossa (the shoulderblade's socket for the round head of the arm bone).

Not all shoulder pain fits into these categories, and TFS will not work for all shoulder problems. Hill–Sachs deformity, acromioclavicular arthritis and fracture don't respond to the maneuver. Nor does frozen shoulder. As I've said repeatedly, it is critical to have an accurate diagnosis before deciding on treatment. Although different diagnostic techniques have variable degrees of accuracy, the definitive diagnostic test for the condition I've mentioned is an MRI. The 1,200 patients I've treated with the TFS have all been diagnosed with MRIs. The instructions below are most successful for shoulder problems that have been diagnosed in that way.

Mastering the TFS

The Triangular Forearm Support isn't difficult or complicated to learn. Most people seem to learn the maneuver quite quickly, but if you don't do yoga, you may need a few attempts. Sometimes one session is enough and the person will have no problem for more than a decade. Other people need to practice the maneuver and then lift their arms daily for weeks or even months. One Hall-of-Fame pitcher had to come up from Pennsylvania to see me three

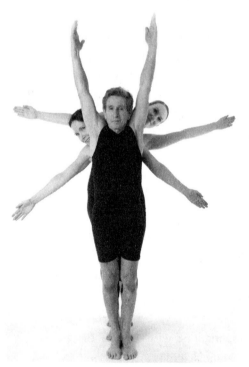

times, but then he got it. Another, a painter of large canvases, came weekly for several months before she was pain-free. But almost everyone with a rotator cuff tear, from a minor rip of fibers to a massive injury in which the tendon is actually torn into two pieces, separated by several centimeters, sees great improvement.

The treatment has two parts. First, you must activate the subscapularis. See the instructions for this below. It takes about 45 seconds to a minute in the correct position to fully activate the muscle, which means you have to hold the position for that length of time. Second, when the subscapularis has been activated, you must stand up and raise your arms to the side quickly and smoothly, without hesitation or fear, until they are straight up with your fingers pointing to the sky. Then immediately lower your arms and raise them again the same way, at least twice. Following that, you must smoothly raise your arms straight out in front of you until they are vertical. Repeat this, too, at least twice. By raising your arms, you are training the activated subscapularis to do the work of the injured supraspinatus.

Be forewarned that raising your injured arm straight up that first time takes courage, because you cannot help but remember the pain you've suffered in the past. You need to be brave and quick to teach the subscapularis its new job—to take over for the supraspinatus. The moment you need the most nerve is when your arm approaches 90 degrees of elevation—the place where it previously began to hurt. At that moment you must act fearlessly and boldly. Do it smoothly, without slowing down, as your arm approaches horizontal. If you don't do it smoothly, the TFS won't work. Do it once, rather quickly, lifting your arms out to the sides all the way up until your fingers are stretched vertically. Then immediately do it again, and again. Then do the same thing, raising your straight arms in front of you smoothly, again and again, all the way to vertical. You are retraining the muscles of the shoulder.

If you have not activated the subscapularis by putting your shoulders into the correct position, the TFS will not work. If you are not sure that you are in the correct position while doing the maneuver, check with a professional—a physical therapist or a yoga therapist—or come to see me. If you find that you are in the correct position with the activated subscapularis and the TFS still does not work after a few tries, it may be time to make sure the original diagnosis was correct, or to check the status of the subscapularis.

THE SECRETS OF TFS SUCCESS

One secret of TFS is reflex inhibition. You cannot feel the subscapularis because it lies beneath the shoulderblade, but you can easily feel the superior third of the trapezius. When the subscapularis is active, the upper trapezius relaxes. When doing the TFS, a friend, teacher or spouse should feel between your shoulderblades and neck to be sure that the trapezius there is totally relaxed and stays that way.

After 45 seconds in the TFS pose, you must emerge from the pose and pretty quickly stand up straight and raise your arms to their full height with the fingers reaching toward the ceiling. Any hesitation will obstruct education of the subscapularis muscle to take over for the injured supraspinatus.

Wall Dog Pose

Benefits and How It Works: Safely reduces pain of arm abduction and flexion by substituting the action of the well-functioning subscapularis muscle for the torn supraspinatus.

Contraindications: Severe adhesive capsulitis, severe injury of the sub-scapularis muscle.

Note: This is the easiest but least effective use of the TFS; still, it works 80 percent of the time.

The Pose: Stand with your feet together facing a wall and about 18 inches from it. Interlock your fingers and press your palms together. The heels of the hands should be touching. Lean forward and rest the little finger sides of your hands and your forearms on the wall in an equilateral triangle at lower chest height. Step two to three feet away from the wall, sliding your forearms another three or four inches down the wall as you do so. Arch your back. Keep your fingers and palms in contact as you press against the wall with your forearms, just below your elbows. Use this pressure to move your shoulders down toward your waist and away from the wall. Enlarge the distance between your shoulders and your ears. The upper third of the trapezius muscle should be soft. The subscapularis should be working, but because it is covered by the shoulderblade, no one can feel it but you. Hold the position for about 45 seconds.

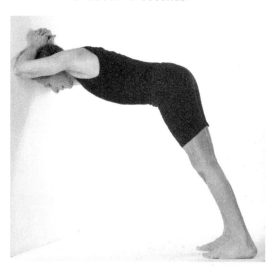

Then stand up and quickly and smoothly raise your arms out to the sides, and in that plane, up above your head, fingers pointing to the ceiling. (Don't go halfway and stop, and don't start by putting your arms out in front of you and raising them in that plane.) Bravely repeat raising your arms at least twice. Then smoothly and quickly raise your arms out in front of you and all the way up, fingers pointing to the ceiling. Do it twice. Avoid raising your arms up halfway, to about where the pain used to start, and stopping there because it has hurt in the past and might hurt now. If you do that, it *will* hurt, and you will have taught yourself nothing. In fact, it will be harder to learn the maneuver after that. Instead, smoothly raise the arms all the way up, and do it rather quickly. This requires nerve, daring, and a certain amount of trust.

Chair Headstand

Benefits and How It Works: Creates a natural gravitational resistance to raising the shoulders away from the ears, activating the subscapularis muscle considerably more than the maneuver against a wall; this is because of the inversion. Resting the legs on a chair reduces the compressive forces on the cervical spine and removes the issue of balance. This is a straightforward headstand, modified for those who are inexperienced. It is the most effective way to activate the subscapularis.

Contraindications: Severe cervical problems, severe vertigo, retinal detachment, glaucoma, orthostatic hypotension. It is ideal for those with mild cervical injuries that make it inadvisable to bear the full weight of the body on the head, but who can withstand the half-weight of their torsos.

Note: It's best to begin practicing this with a teacher or other spotter.

The Pose: Place the back of a chair against a wall so it doesn't slide. If the chair is not upholstered, place a folded yoga mat or blanket on the seat

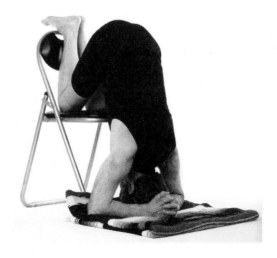

to cushion your knees. Stand on a blanket folded in four with the backs of your knees against the front of the chair. Raise your right knee and place it on the seat of the chair. Your right shin should be vertical, rising up from the chair. Bend forward, placing both palms on the floor. Lift the left leg behind you, resting your bent knee on the seat of the chair, shin vertical. Walk your hands in toward the front of the chair, so your torso is close to vertical. Bend your elbows slowly until the top of your head—not your forehead—rests firmly on the blanket. Interlock your fingers, with your palms against one another behind your head. Press down with your elbows and the first four or five inches of your forearms just below your elbows to raise your shoulders away from your ears. When you are stable, walk your knees out toward the front edge of the seat of the chair to orient your torso more vertically. Hold yourself there for 45 seconds. Then come down quickly by bringing first one knee (or foot) to the floor, then the other. Quickly stand up. Immediately lift both arms smoothly and rather quickly toward the ceiling.

If getting right up makes you dizzy or you tend to stagger, then do the headstand for a little longer, say a minute or more, and get up more slowly, with someone helping you. If you continue to do inversions in this or just about any way, your sympathetic nervous system will soon learn to contract the smaller blood vessels of your legs when you get up, and the lightheadedness will either vanish or greatly subside. In the meantime, you can stand with the backs of your knees against the front of the chair to stabilize yourself as you raise your arms.

Sirsasana
Headstand

Benefits and How It Works: This is another good way to activate the subscapularis, provided balance is not an issue.

Warning: Always use a blanket placed on the floor six inches from a wall to help prevent falling backward. Get the approval of a qualified teacher before doing headstand without a wall behind you.

Contraindications: Imbalance, glaucoma, Chiari malformation, cerebral aneurysm or other cerebrovascular problems, herniated cervical disc, cervical facet syndrome, severe hypertension, orthostatic hypotension, history of head, neck or brain surgery, frozen shoulder, retinal detachment.

The Pose: Place a folded blanket on the floor with one edge against a wall. Kneel on the floor nine inches away from its edge. Clasp your hands firmly and rest them in the middle of the blanket to form two sides of an equilateral triangle. Place the top of your head (not your forehead) in the middle of the triangle. Straighten your knees and slowly walk in toward your head, until your pelvis is over your arms and head. Then gradually lift your legs to vertical. After your balance is secure, press downward with your elbows and forearms and lift your shoulders far away from the floor. Keep your head on the blanket. Remain in this position for 45 seconds. Then slowly lower your legs, kneel, stand up and proceed at once to raising your arms as described above.

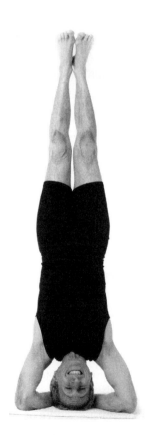

CHAPTER TEN

Headache

L IKE SO MANY other medical conditions, headache is a symptom rather than a diagnosis, and should be treated after the cause is known. Your headache might be due to stress, to a problem with your sinuses, to high blood pressure or even to having not eaten lunch. Some sources say there are over 200 types of headache, from harmless to life-threatening. And, according to the National Headache Foundation, nearly three-quarters of people who have headaches have more than one type.

Consultation with a physician is indicated if you're over fifty and experiencing a headache that feels different from any you've had before, if you're confused or are awakened during the night by pain. Any change in your vision, a headache that gets worse when you cough or chew, a very stiff neck and/or fever are reasons to consult your doctor, and that's also true if you have been diagnosed with HIV, cancer or thrombosis. Please be mindful: a really severe headache calls for medical attention.

In some cases, such as migraine, tension and cervicogenic headache (headache originating in your neck), medications are the standard treatment: over-the-counter pain relievers, and substances only your doctor can prescribe. If your headache is not a symptom of a treatable underlying condition, I believe that yoga can help, and research confirms that.[1]

Migraines, tension headaches and cervicogenic headaches are the most responsive to yoga. If yours is a tension headache, the chapter on depression is for you because it contains information on how to de-stress. See the chapter on PMS for headache that seems to occur at a specific time of the month as it could be linked to hormones, and if your teeth or face hurt in addition to your headache, refer to the chapter on colds and sinus problems.

Headache Triggers

There are as many as fifty triggers for various types of headache, and some of them apply across the board.[2] These include female hormones, fatigue, sunlight, certain foods and substances (such as caffeine and the nitrates in some processed foods) and odors, according to the Handbook for Clinical Neurology.[3] Ironically, judicious use of caffeine can also help relieve a headache under some circumstances.

It's a good idea to observe yourself to discover what things trigger your headaches, and then to avoid them whenever possible. There is yoga to do if you know you're prone to headaches during your menstrual cycle, but apart from birth control and doses of testosterone there is little you can do to control the relevant hormones. You can, however, take charge of things like getting enough sleep, staying away from food triggers like aged cheese or red wine and when you drink alcohol, do it with moderation.

Tension Headache

The National Headache Foundation did a survey that showed tension-type headaches were the second most common after migraine.[4] A tension-type headache can be an occasional thing or it can be chronic, especially for women. It can vary in frequency and intensity. Stress and fatigue can be factors, and so can depression or ongoing physical problems. Some believe depression to be an important cause.[5]

The symptoms of a tension headache are mild to moderate and are probably caused by activity in the brain and the muscles of the face, neck and head. Symptoms include a feeling of tightness—some describe it as a vise-like band around their heads—muscle stiffness, pressure or diffuse pain. For many the pain goes on without a feeling of throbbing. Most people feel a dull ache in the forehead, temples or back of the head and neck on both sides. If your headache is related to anxiety, you may experience insomnia, and if it's due in part to depression you may wake several times during the night. Though a lot of research has been done on the physical mechanisms of tension-type headaches, there is still work to be done. Usual medical treatments include over-the-counter painkillers and caffeine.[6]

Migraine Headache

More than 29.5 million Americans suffer from migraine, and women are three times more likely to have these types of headaches than men, according to the National Headache Association. Women in middle age or who are perimenopausal are the group most likely to be affected, along with those in households at the lower end of the income scale.[7] Migraine often runs in families and may be hereditary.

Some of the symptoms of migraine are well known: pain usually occurs on one side of the head and feels as if it's pulsing or throbbing. Four out of ten patients (39 percent) say migraine drives them to their beds, frequently for days at a time. In 1998 Americans spent 112 million days in bed because of migraine headaches. Medical treatments have probably reduced that enormous number. One reason people take to their beds is that bright lights and loud sounds increase their discomfort, and the bedroom is relatively quiet and dark. Visual disturbances are typical with migraine, and physical activity such as climbing stairs can worsen the pain. Nausea and vomiting are not uncommon. I have a friend whose migraine headache usually brings on vomiting, after which the headache dissipates.

As many as 20 percent of those who get migraines experience an aura, which occurs before the headache itself hits and may serve as a warning. These visual disturbances are due to short-term changes in the activity of nerve cells. They may see zigzagging lines, dots, flashing lights. They may have blind spots in their field of vision, tingling in the arm or face and confused speech. These symptoms of migraine are emotionally as well as physically upsetting; poses for relaxation, as well as those specifically for migraine, should help.

When brain cells become agitated, they cause the trigeminal nerve to emit chemicals that inflame and swell blood vessels on the surface of the brain. These swollen vessels telegraph pain signals to the brain stem, which processes them and sends them out. The person with a migraine usually feels the pain around the eyes and/or temple, face, jaw or neck. The whole head can feel so sensitive it can be painful even to shave or brush your hair.

An analysis done by the University of Alabama Headache Treatment and Research Program found that emotional stress, disrupted sleep patterns and various odors were major migraine triggers, and that headaches associated with female hormones and menstruation were more severe, lasted longer and were harder to treat than some other migraines.[8] Dr. Adam Hamawy, a plastic surgeon in Manhattan, does a relatively simple procedure with botulinim toxin that is said to be nearly 90 percent effective.

Cervicogenic Headache

Though there has been some controversy about the existence of cervicogenic headache, I am a believer that when something pathological is going on in the many small structures of the neck, it can cause the head to ache. Laboratory and clinical studies have confirmed that pain from upper cervical joints and muscles can be referred to the head, according to an article published in *Lancet Neurology*,[9] and I often see patients who have this type of headache. Usually the muscles in the neck go into spasm, and since they connect pretty closely and coordinate with muscles in the scalp and head, pain results.

In my opinion, the biggest causes of cervicogenic headache are degenerative joint disease (arthritis) and problems with posture. Your head weighs between 14 and 18 pounds—as much or more than a bowling ball. People tend to bend forward at the computer, in conversation, when reading or watching TV and when driving. Our chairs have curves in them that conspire to get us to lean forward. Just being interested in something is often enough to make a person's upper body tilt toward the person or object. Just think about it. If you held a bowling ball out from your torso with your arm for as long as you sit at the computer or watch TV or commute, you wouldn't be surprised when your arm began to hurt. It's the same when the weight of your head pulls you toward something or someone. Obviously one way to prevent posture-based cervicogenic headaches is simply to change your posture. Open your chest, by which I mean the place between your nipples and collarbones. When you do this, you should feel the little muscles in your back contracting and the muscles of your neck relax. Your head will of necessity move back until it is balanced above your shoulders.

Sitting at the computer, looking at the screen, is not a natural posture. It's not the distance at which you have a conversation even with a close friend or any circumstance that isn't intimate. That distance at which you focus on your computer screen has been described as "computer distance" by Mary Pullig Schatz, a physician and noted yoga teacher, therapist and author. If you feel that you're leaning forward in a way that could affect the muscles and joints in your neck while you're working at your computer, it might not be a bad idea to get glasses that are geared to helping you see at a greater distance to help you correct your posture.

Arthritis can develop in the neck because of the way nature has constructed it, with little or no extra room. The joints are close to the openings where nerves exit the spinal cord, and the nerves have very little wiggle room if there is any narrowing of the joints due to arthritis or inflammation. We physicians can't do much apart from medication for swelling of joints; your body can do more by itself, using a molecule called PGC-1alpha. This is a potent endogenous anti-inflammatory that reduces swelling anywhere it occurs in the human body. Gentle activities such as yoga and tai chi, and especially yoga done for long periods of time, encourage the body to release this miraculous substance from your muscles.

Even when swelling and pain persist, there are ways you can work with yoga cleverly. Many yoga poses will help with posture, both sitting and standing. Not all of them are included here because of space constraints, but you will find others in chapter 9 of my book with Ellen Saltonstall, *Yoga for Arthritis* (the chapter on the cervical spine).

A third condition that occurs in the neck isn't as common, but if you've had it or even if you've seen it on someone else, you won't forget it. It's called spastic torticollis—literally, spasmodic turning of the neck. It happens when one group of muscles gets really tight and turns the neck. Sometimes the head turns in jerking motions, and sometimes it turns and stays in an unnatural place. Matsyendrasana (p. 42) is helpful, as is just about any twisting pose. This is a condition so painful and so intransigent that you may need a yoga therapist or a doctor who can give an injection that will alleviate it at least temporarily. Yoga can be invaluable, obviating the injection, or converting its effect from temporary to permanent.

Appropriate yoga is good for almost anything that ails the neck and for pain referred from the neck to the head. Basically it's a question of motor learning, whether for posture or for arthritis. It improves the suppleness of the neck muscles and increases the versatility of the joints so they can move more easily in many different ways. It refines the coordination of the various muscle groups so muscles aren't pulling against each other with such ferocity. And lastly, yoga facilitates relaxation in the neck as it does elsewhere.

A First Cousin of Setu Bandhasana
Out On the Table or Chair Pose

This is a yoga-like pose that I saw Mr. Iyengar use many times. On one such occasion, the student had just arrived and had acquired a terrible headache while traveling. After staying in this posture for ten minutes, he got up and said softly, "It's gone." Mr. Iyengar laughed and said, "No one could keep a headache after that!"

Mr. Iyengar kept a vigilant eye on that person throughout the period of extension described below, and I strongly recommend that this pose be done at first with a trustworthy partner. The stretch has to be gradual and adapted to your neck to be used safely.

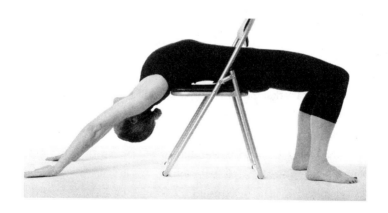

Benefits and How It Works: By stretching the body's ventral muscles, the facial and cranial musculature is prompted to relax.

Helpful Hints: Arching the lower thoracic and upper lumbar spine can be painful. Keep them as close as possible to the table or chair.

Contraindications: Cerebral, carotid or vertebral arterial aneurysm, cervical stenosis, grade II or higher cervical antero- or retrolisthesis.

The Pose: Use a firm couch, a sturdy table, or a chair covered with a blanket at one end to blunt the edge. Place a chair beyond that edge, facing the table or the other chair.

Lie on your back, head and upper shoulders off the edge of the couch or table or chair. Have your helper sit in the (other) chair and hold your head up. The helper gradually lowers your head, stretching it gently from your shoulders; when your neck is extended to 45 degrees, wait about a minute and a half. Then raise your arms over your head so your hands are on either side of the helper's arms, palms up.

After 30 seconds in this position, bend your knees and push yourself a small amount further off the table, or inch forward on the chair as the helper slowly lowers your head a little bit further. Continue in one-inch increments every 30 seconds until the lower third of your shoulderblades reaches the edge of the table or chair. At this point, your head and arms will be inclining even further downward. Stay in this position for another minute or two, letting gravity stretch the muscles of your abdomen, chest and throat. Then your helper and you together should lift your head and arms back to a supine position. Rest there for a few moments before sitting up.

Setu Bandhasana
Bridge Pose

Benefits and How It Works: Contracting the middle and lower back, stretching the ventral musculature and breathing as above seems to restore the cerebral circulation and relax the muscles of the scalp.

Contraindications: Carotid dissection or other carotid arterial or jugular venous pathology, cervical disc herniation.

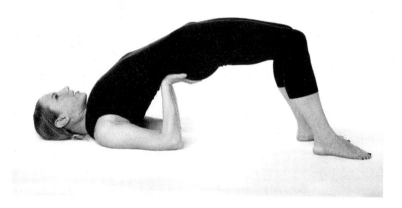

Helpful Hints: The further you pull your shoulders away from your head and toward your hips, the more effective this posture will be.

The Pose: Lie supine on a mat, arms at your sides, a second mat folded beneath your shoulders. Bend your knees. Do not move your feet as you inhale, but push them away from you as you raise your torso off the mat. In other words, straighten your knees a little without sliding your feet away from you. The action will raise your chest forward, toward a position over your throat.

Place your hands, fingers pointing toward each other, under the back of your waist. After you establish stability in this position, press your feet away from you, again without moving them. Use this force to raise your torso higher and lift your chest more vertically up over your chin. Breathe slowly and symmetrically. Fill the bottoms of your lungs first, then the middle, stretching them out to the sides and in toward each other. Then inflate the very tops of the lungs, between your shoulders and your throat.

Do not count the breaths; rather, breathe until you are comfortable. Stop before you are uncomfortable. Come out of the pose by reversing the steps above: relax the pressure on the feet and release your hands and slowly unroll the torso. Remain with knees bent for a short time before extending your legs and sitting up. Other versions are on pages 61 and 62.

Paschimottanasana
Seated Forward Bend Pose

Benefits and How It Works: Stretching the hamstrings generates impulses from the golgi tendon organs that tend to relax the extensor muscles of the entire trunk, neck and scalp. This effect begins within 90 seconds of entering the pose.

Contraindications: Severe osteoporosis, herniated lumbar intervertebral disc, late pregnancy, severe impingement syndrome (shoulder).

Helpful Hints: Many people believe the point of this pose is to bring their heads to their shins, but that is just a by-product of the pose. Think of your navel descending down between your thighs. *Paschimottan* means "extreme bend of the west." Yogis classically face east when they do asana, so the attention here is on the back of the body.

The Pose: Sit upright on a soft blanket, knees fully extended, ankles together. Elongate your torso vertically as you inhale. Arch your back slightly. Exhale as you draw your entire torso forward, hinging at the hips, not the waist. As you lean forward, turn your hands downward and outward, grasping one wrist with the opposite hand beyond your feet. Flex the quadriceps and outer thigh to inactivate the hamstrings and muscles of the inner thigh.

Rest your cheekbones on your shins, urging your head and shoulders forward, not down. Clasp the wrist tightly, but relax the arms and shoulders. Let your elbows pull you forward and down until your chin is on your legs, just below your knees. Breathe quietly. To leave the pose, unclasp your hands and slowly rise to the upright position.

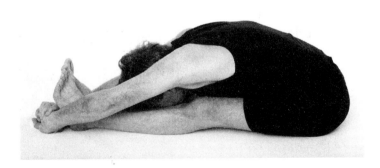

LESS CHALLENGING VARIATION:

Use a belt around the middle of the soles of the feet to pull yourself forward, not down. Retain a slightly arched back throughout. Extending the knees maximally is important to set up the proper reflex inhibition of hamstring contraction, as well as to initiate the basic effect on headache.

Viparita Karani
Inclined Plane Pose

Benefits and How It Works: The slight inversion distributes the blood more to the upper body and less to the lower. This changes gravity's tug on the large and small blood vessels of the upper torso, neck and head. Recalibrating the tension of the tiny muscles of the arterioles often relieves tension and migraine headaches.

Contraindications: Extreme hypertension, aneurysm or cerebral clips.

Helpful Hints: Lying at too great an angle in this pose can actually increase your pain. It's best to elevate the torso to 35 degrees and then silently scan your body from head to toe for sensations. Do this for as long as you stay in the pose, scanning from head to toe and then back up again. Do not neglect the neck, throat, face and head.

The Pose: Lie supine with your legs and torso on an inclining stack of pillows or bolsters, or a slant board covered with a soft towel or blanket. The optimal angle is 35 degrees. Your head should be horizontal. Let your facial expression dissolve.

You may stay for 5 to 15 minutes.

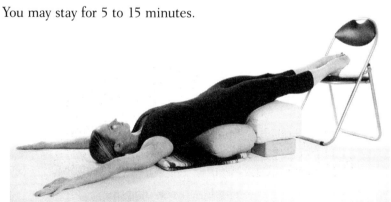

CHAPTER ELEVEN

Weight Control

Have you noticed that almost all the yogis you see in online photos and yoga classes are slim? That's just one of the factors adding to the common misconception that by just doing yoga you will lose weight or prevent pounds from piling on.

In his book *The Science of Yoga*, William Broad accurately observed that while aerobic exercise quickens the metabolism and is beneficial for weight loss, yoga slows metabolism—the opposite of the action needed to burn off fat. I know that is true, but I think there is more to the story. Hatha yoga is definitely an activity, and any activity can burn calories. Some yoga types—ashtanga, for example—are more active than other types. If you're doing a strenuous, active practice, it certainly can be almost aerobic and can quicken the metabolism. Many schools of yoga, however, emphasize holding a pose rather than moving through it, and ask students to pay attention to alignment rather than motion. Still, for several reasons I don't think it's an accident that a majority of serious yoga practitioners are well within normal weight limits.

Many yoga poses stretch the stomach lining, which is a weight-limiting factor. This is confusing: for many, the idea of stretching the stomach suggests making it bigger and creating more room inside for food. That's not what I'm talking about. The stomach has stretch receptors that report to the appetite centers in the brain via the vagus nerve. When you stimulate the stretch receptors in the stomach, the signals tell the appetite centers that enough is enough. These transient stretches will do nothing to enlarge the capacity of the stomach. On the contrary, they will make you feel fuller and thereby decrease the amount you eat.

It is not clear whether all mammals have this system, and many animals such as horses are constrained by low-calorie food sources to eat virtually all the time. Some say that we humans have developed culture partially because we can quickly obtain all the sustenance we need and then have time to do things other than eat.

Many factors contribute to the tendency to put on weight. Some of us inherit a body type that's likely to become chunky. Others just can't stay away from sweets or carbs or processed foods. Let's face it, weight control isn't necessarily easy, particularly if you're born into a family where many members have big butts or big bellies, or who regularly gather in the kitchen and eat, especially when something stressful has happened. A daughter's chance of being obese is affected by something totally beyond her control—her mother's weight during pregnancy.[1] And as we know, some women have trouble shedding pounds after giving birth. It's not surprising that personality traits such as impulsiveness have a role in being overweight.

But we don't lack energy when it comes to trying to change our outward shape. Just about every diet imaginable exists, along with some that are hard to imagine. There's the cabbage soup diet, the Zone, Weight Watchers, the South Beach Diet, the Atkins high-protein diet. A friend of mine developed her own weight-loss program. She ate nothing but oranges for two weeks and did lose several pounds. Many of us have tried high-protein diets to lose weight quickly. My neighbor even emptied the refrigerator and tried having high-protein, low-calorie dinners delivered every night. I go along with the National Institutes of Health: the best weight-loss plan controls caloric intake but allows you to eat all foods within reason.

It's well known that many Hindus in India are vegetarians, and I wondered if that helped keep their weight healthy. It turns out that research on this has been published, assessing forty research papers that studied the relationship between diet and body mass.[2] Female vegetarians weigh 6–17 percent less than their counterparts who eat meat; male vegetarians weighed 8–17 percent less. Vegans, who eat no meat or dairy products, were thinner yet. And it's well documented that vegetarians are healthier than the general population, and less subject to type 2 diabetes, hypertension and cancer.

The best way to lose weight and keep off the extra pounds is to do it slowly but surely. If you lose one or two pounds a week consistently until you have reached your goal, you'll have a better chance of avoiding the immediate gain that leads to yo-yo dieting. Being overweight is a source of shame for many, and some people give up trying to lose pounds to avoid more shame—the shame of failure. One stereotype I've encountered is that fat people are lazy, but some of the most vigorous, hardworking and energetic people I've encountered in my life are significantly overweight.

There is a lot of research being done about the effects of yoga on weight control, partially because of the obesity epidemic that is leading to increased health risks and health costs, but as of today there is no definitive proof that yoga is beneficial for those who need to lose weight or are trying to avoid putting on pounds. However, a couple of studies suggest there will be increasing evidence in favor of yoga. A study of 15,550 adults aged fifty-three to fifty-seven years old concluded that regular yoga practice over a period of years was associated with reduced weight gain, especially for those who were overweight. The study authors acknowledged that they could not infer that yoga caused this result, and more study is necessary, but their work points in a positive direction.[3]

Yoga is helpful for weight control because it increases your confidence and sense of well-being, and it contributes to better overall bodily health. It's grounding and steadying and therefore improves impulse control. In addition, it promotes body awareness—awareness not only of the foods we're eating but of how much of those foods we're putting in. That contributes to making better decisions about what to eat. Since losing weight is dependent on consuming fewer calories, increased awareness is helpful. Judi Bar, Yoga Program Director at the Cleveland Clinic, participated in writing a July 2013 study in the *American Journal of Lifestyle Medicine* emphasizing this point, and added that yoga can help in general by lessening back and joint pain to allow increased activity.[4]

My own diet plan for overweight patients—the plan I give them before recommending yoga that will stretch their stomachs and help them cut down on their food intake and also help their inner selves—goes like this:

Eat anything you want, as much as you want, *but stop eating while you're still a little hungry, say 5–10 percent*. You can lose weight this way if you just push the chair away from the table a few minutes earlier than you usually would.

When you leave the table a little hungry, a feedback loop takes effect. The food you've eaten goes to your stomach and gets digested, then the glucose that's produced by the digestive processes reaches your brain and turns off the appetite center. If you leave the table a little hungry, an hour to an hour and a half later those hunger pangs will be gone. It's the same idea as when you were a kid and your mother didn't want you to eat too many cookies an hour before dinner because it would ruin your appetite, only this time limiting your appetite is your goal.

Yoga fits right in by stimulating the stretch receptors in our stomachs, helping to modify the appetite and druglessly curtailing caloric input. That strategy has been successful with a number of my patients, particularly when combined with a little explanation. It requires some self-discipline, but you feel good, a little lighter and more mobile right away, and soon living with the very slight hunger gets to be a pleasant habit that helps you lose a few pounds a month—slow weight loss that helps you keep the extra pounds off. Best of all, six months later, when you've lost quite a lot, the stomach is smaller, and the combination of earlier satiety and the enhanced stretch response will help you stay that way.

Here are three poses to stimulate the stomach's stretch receptors. Do them about a half hour to an hour before meals. And, of course, on an empty stomach.

Virabhadrasana I and/or III
Warrior I/III Pose

Benefits and How It Works: The pose stimulates the stretch receptors in the stomach and the closer sections of the duodenum, sending inhibiting signals to the appetite centers in the brain along vagal afferent nerve fibers.

Contraindications: Recent abdominal surgery, moderate or severe spinal stenosis, severe hypertension.

The Pose: Stand or jump your legs four and a half feet apart, arms horizontal, palms down. Take two breaths. Turn the left foot 90 degrees outward and the right 30 degrees inward as you raise your arms to vertical. With your legs

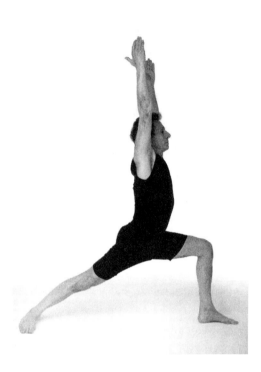

straight, swivel your hips so that your navel is facing the same direction as your forward foot. Bend your left knee to a right angle, shin vertical, thigh horizontal. Stretch your fingers and especially your thumbs up to the sky. Breathe evenly for 60 seconds. Return to standing by reversing the sequence.

This is Virabhadrasana I (Warrior I). To go on to Virabhadrasana III, bend the forward knee and incline your torso forward, keeping your back straight. Then launch upward and forward as you straighten the right knee and raise the left leg to horizontal. Stretch from heel to fingertips, especially the backs of the hands. Look straight ahead. Stay aloft for up to 30 seconds, then reverse the steps, return your foot to the mat and repeat on the other side.

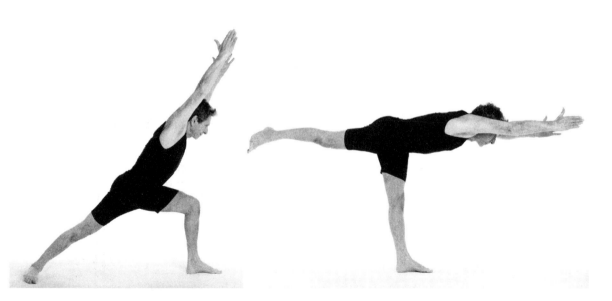

VARIATIONS FOR VIRABHADRASANA I:

1. Place the thigh of your bent leg on a chair seat. Place one hand on the bent thigh; use the other for balance by holding the chair back. As you get more secure, work to raise yourself off the chair. Use your legs, not your arms, to do this. Keep your arms at your sides or raise them.

2. Place a block under the forward leg. This lifts the torso and rocks it backward, encouraging more extension of the lower lumbar spine. Beginning the pose with a wider stance, in which the legs are not in a straight line, enhances the therapeutic effects of this pose.

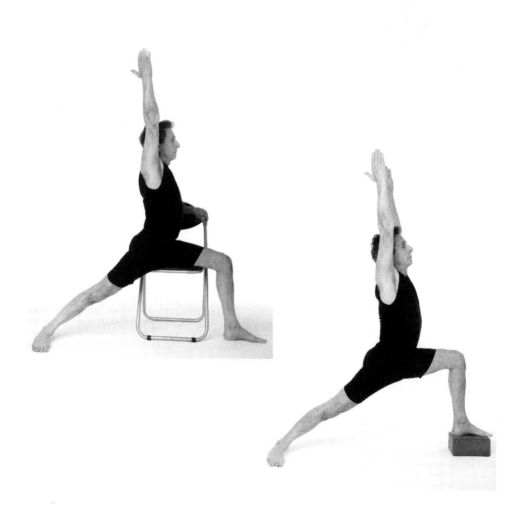

VARIATION FOR VIRABHADRASANA III:

Supplement your balance by resting your outstretched hands on the back of a chair about 18 inches in front of you. Fingers point forward, palms face each other.

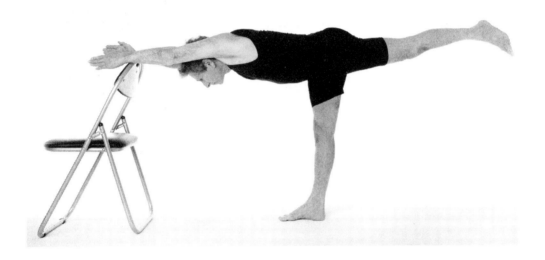

Padahasthasana
Hands to Feet Pose

Benefits and How It Works: Stretches the stomach toward the head, toward the feet and sideways. If your back stays straight, your chest moves away from your abdomen, and the esophagus tugs on the top of the stomach, while the relative anchoring of the intestine by the mesentery holds the bottom of the stomach and the duodenum downward. The pressure of the folded abdomen on the stomach stretches it sideways. These pressures lower appetite.

Contraindications: Plantar fasciitis, osteoporosis, hamstring tear, severe disc herniation, ischial bursitis.

Helpful Hints: Bend forward from your hips as though they were hinges and the only moving parts. If you can place your hands under the soles of your feet, pull upward—not inward—by putting pressure on the balls of your feet with your palms. As you pull, bend your elbows out to the side, not toward your shins.

The Pose: Stand erect with feet parallel, hands at your sides. Take a good breath and as you exhale, descend your straight torso until it is flush against your thighs, hands under your forefeet, palms up. Gently and symmetrically bend your elbows out to the side, drawing your cheeks and chin downward. Do not move your feet, but smoothly and increasingly pull them outward (without their moving) using that effort to stretch and relax the adductors, and maintain your weight equally on all parts of both feet.

LESS CHALLENGING VARIATION:

Place palms, wrists, then elbows on the front of the seat of a chair, descending gradually further over time. Be sure to keep your back straight.

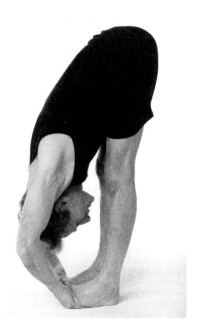

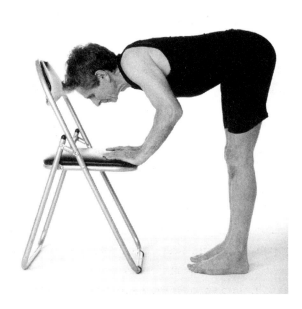

Ardha Matsyendrasana I
Seated Half Twist Pose

Benefits and How It Works: Twists the stomach clockwise and counterclockwise, reducing appetite, giving a sense of lightness. By carrying the top of the stomach to the side and retaining the intestines in a more or less neutral position, the stomach revolves at least a quarter turn.

Contraindications: Severe herniated disc, severe scoliosis, kyphosis or spondylolisthesis, large ventral hernia, shoulder derangement.

Helpful Hints: Sit in a stable position so your support is not disturbed by the actions of getting into the pose. Lift your torso up from the abdomen as far as you comfortably can.

The Pose: Sit, bending your right knee so your thigh is flat against the floor and your right foot is close to your left buttock. Place the left foot high up against the outer right thigh, sole flat on the floor. Raise your right arm over your left knee as you twist to the left, sliding your right armpit over

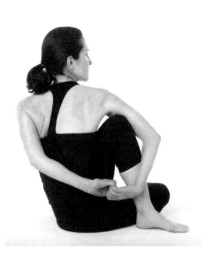

the left knee. Walk your left hand behind yourself counterclockwise as you bend your right elbow and seek your left hand with your right until the left hand clasps the right behind your back. Retract your left shoulder back counterclockwise to reach your left hand further behind you. Also retract your right shoulder, using the shoulderblade to impel your right upper ribs and chest forward and to the left. Raise your entire chest off the base of your buttocks, thighs and lumbar spine. Look straight ahead or out over your left shoulder.

VARIATIONS:

1. One variation keeps the right arm straight, possibly tucked in between the left foot and the right thigh. In this case the left hand supplies more support, and helps you raise your chest away from your abdomen.

2. The simplest useful variation is to start by sitting in a chair or armchair,

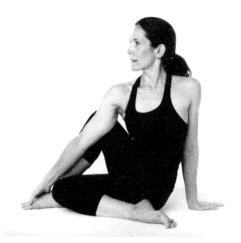
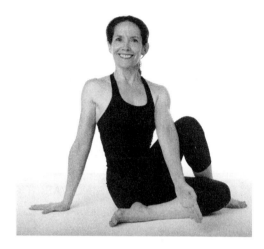

feet flat on the floor. Hold the left side or arm of the chair with your right hand; stretch your left arm back around the chair to the right edge of the backrest or the right arm of the chair. Pull your left shoulder back, and urge your right chest forward, especially the lowest ribs. Make your spine as long as possible.

Jathara Parivartasana
Revolved Abdomen Pose

Benefits and How It Works: This pose stimulates stretch receptors in the stomach and esophagus from top to bottom and also from side to side. The digestive organs are transiently but dramatically stretched when the chest is stabilized and the legs are maximally lowered off to the side.

Contraindications: Recent gastrointestinal surgery, including the gall bladder, pancreas and liver, recently herniated disc, severe arthritis at the thoracolumbar junction (T12–L1). Because the spine is held in place by gravity, this pose is safer in scoliosis, kyphosis and spondylolisthesis.

The Pose: Lie supine, arms stretched out at 90 degrees to the torso, palms up. Breathe in as you lengthen your fingertips away from your shoulders. Exhale, making your abdomen thin as you raise your bent legs and straighten them as they come to vertical. Extend your heels up as high as possible. Inhale as you tilt your hips to the right by moving your buttocks a few inches to the left. This will enable you to keep your ankles together as you exhale and lower both legs together to the right, so they make a right angle with your pelvis and torso. Your left chest will have a tendency to rise up as your legs descend. Counter this by pressing the back of the right hand down onto the floor to keep the left back ribs against the floor. Lengthen your torso from coccyx to the top of your head again, breathing quietly for at least 30 seconds. Then raise your legs back to vertical, tilt to the left by moving the buttocks slightly to the right, and repeat the descent on the left side.

LESS CHALLENGING VARIATIONS:

Legs can be bent at first. Blocks and bolsters can limit the legs' sideways descent when you begin. The knees can actually be used as a kind of rheostat: as you improve in the pose, as your joints become more mobile, you can straighten the legs more, which will strengthen the stimulus on the esophageal and gastric stretch receptors by increasing forces on them.

Other Poses for Weight Control: Setu Bandhasana (p. 60), Parivrtta Trikonasana (p. 78), Parivrtta Parsvakonasana (p. 81), Parivrtta Ardha Chandrasana (p. 93).

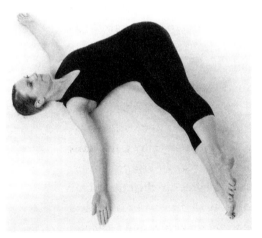
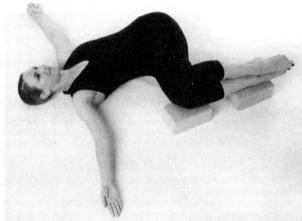

CHAPTER TWELVE

Common Cold

I'S NOT SURPRISING that virtually all children under the age of five are exposed to viruses that cause the common cold, or that the stuffy nose and headache—the misery—often recur in people of all ages.[1] I never gave it much thought, and maybe just assumed that the common cold (or upper respiratory tract infection, URI) had been around forever. Not so, according to the Society for General Microbiology.[2] One of the main viruses that cause colds—the human metapneumovirus—was discovered in 2001; it had probably been circulating in humans for at least half a century, and most likely had been around in other life forms for about 200 years. Most surprising to me is that this common cold virus crossed the species barrier from birds. Who would have thought the Kleenex-consuming common cold originated in our fine feathered friends?

I've wondered, sometimes, while blowing my nose, why the cold is called a cold. One possibility is that before people understood viruses caused illness, they thought just being cold could make you sick. Another is that according to the ancient theory of humors, phlegm was associated with winter. From my own observation, it does seem that people get more colds in the winter and spring, possibly because of more viral activity and distribution, possibly because contagion is increased as we tend to be more crowded indoors in the colder winter months and early spring. However, considering urban mass transport and climate change, we may be just as contagion-prone all year long, and frigid air conditioning lowers temperatures as much as some warmer winters.[3]

When you have a cold, you probably have a stuffy or runny nose, a sneeze, cough, sore throat or headache. One of the main differences between a cold and the flu is that with flu, fever is often present. Here's a rule of thumb if you're trying to figure out which you have: if it's above the neck, it's a cold. If your symptoms are below the neck—chest congestion, muscle aches and pains, fever—you're more likely to have the flu. A cold virus spreads through tiny air droplets that are released when infected persons sneeze, cough or blow their noses. You can catch a cold from a person who sneezes while passing by you or from a friend who recently borrowed your pen and left virus particles there that easily can be transferred by your hand to your nose, mouth or eye. Hand sanitizers have recently been shown to be poor at preventing colds, but thorough hand washing for at least 20 seconds does radically cut down on the number of virus particles.

Popular cold treatments for symptomatic relief include over-the-counter antihistamines, cough medicines and decongestants. There is some scientific evidence that combination products containing these three substances are helpful for adults.[4] Some other preventatives and remedies are also at least somewhat effective. If you do catch a cold, drink lots of fluids and rest.

Vitamin C

For more than sixty years vitamin C has been considered by some to be capable of preventing, relieving and shortening the duration of the common cold. In 2007 the *Cochrane Reviews* looked at many studies that included 11,077 participants over a number of years, to see if taking 200 milligrams of vitamin C a day could reduce the incidence, severity or duration of colds.

The reviewers concluded that vitamin C supplements taken as a preventative don't reduce the number of colds for most. But there was evidence that preventative doses of the vitamin might help those who exercise strenuously for short periods of time or who linger in cold environments. A small but statistically significant benefit in shortening the duration and severity of colds shows that vitamin C does play a role in the body's defense mechanisms.

Zinc

Some of my friends find that a combination of zinc gluconate lozenges and hot green tea shortens the duration of a cold and lessens its misery. A randomized, double-blind, placebo-controlled 1996 study backs them up, having found that the formulated 13.1 milligram dose of zinc studied significantly reduced the duration of a cold when used within twenty-four hours of the onset of symptoms, though how it works remains unknown. Some people object to the taste of zinc gluconate lozenges.[5] There are many different products containing zinc, all of which may not be equally effective. Doses of zinc used in various studies have ranged widely in quantity, but a recommended dose is not greater than 75 milligrams per day during the symptoms of the cold, according to a 2013 article in the *Cochrane Review*. Further research is needed to see if there is a benefit from using zinc as a preventative. However, according to the Mayo Clinic, intranasal zinc can damage a person's sense of smell, perhaps permanently.[6]

As far as I know, there has been no research into the effectiveness of yoga for treating the common cold. The poses I give below are, I believe, helpful, but my proof is anecdotal. Still, I am absolutely sure that doing yoga has helped many patients, and it makes me feel better when I have a cold.

Research has shown that yoga may boost the immune system. In a groundbreaking study, some participants spent two weeks doing yoga that included asana, breathing exercises and meditation, while others went on nature walks or listened to music. Blood samples showed a change in gene expression that suggests yoga can boost immunities. Those who did non-yoga activities had changes in the expression of thirty-eight genes called peripheral blood mononuclear cells. In comparison, yoga produced changes in 111 of these circulating cells.[7] This suggests to me that a comprehensive yoga practice can help people fight off some infections, possibly including colds.

In the first class that I attended with B. K. S. Iyengar in India, students did the headstand. I thought I was prepared, as I had done that and every other pose in his book *Light on Yoga* many times. But with famous Iyengar strictness, he came over to me while I was upside down, punched my stomach and said, "This, what you're doing, is not my yoga." He was deft. The blow didn't topple me or knock the wind out of me, but I will never forget it. My headstand had been an inverted version of Little Lord Fauntleroy: backside and belly sticking out equally egregiously in opposite directions.

Some friends and fellow yogis question doing the headstand for a cold. They argue that inversion makes their noses stuffier or runnier, increases congestion and in general makes them more miserable. I find that it allows all the congestion to flow away from me. After a few minutes of headstand I always feel better and breathe more easily.

Sirsasana
Headstand

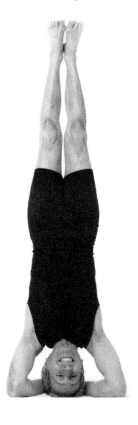

Benefits and How It Works: I believe inversion for about five minutes raises the venous pressure in the capillaries of the nose, sinuses and throat. When you are upright again, these vessels react by contracting, substantially reducing congestion.

Warning: Always use a blanket placed on the floor six inches from a wall to help prevent falling backward. Get the approval of a qualified teacher before doing headstand without a wall behind you.

Contraindications: Imbalance, glaucoma, Chiari malformation, cerebral aneurysm or other cerebrovascular problems, herniated cervical disc, cervical facet syndrome, severe hypertension, orthostatic hypotension, history of head, neck or brain surgery, frozen shoulder, retinal detachment.

The Pose: Place a folded blanket on the floor against a wall and kneel on the floor nine inches away from its edge. Clasp your hands firmly and rest them in the middle of the blanket to form two sides of an equilateral triangle. Place the top of your head (not your forehead) in the middle of the triangle. Straighten your knees and slowly walk in toward your head, until your pelvis is over your arms and head. Then gradually lift your legs to vertical. After your balance is secure, press downward with your elbows and forearms and lift your shoulders away from the floor. Keep your head on the blanket. Remain in this position for 45 seconds. Then slowly lower your legs, kneel, and stand up.

VARIATION:

If you cannot do headstand, see the chapter on rotator cuff injury (p. 101) for ways to achieve a similar effect.

Uttanasana
Standing Forward Bend Pose

Benefits and How It Works: Helps clear stuffy nose and ease congestion. This pose combines the self-induced vascular congestion that inverted postures produce with intense hamstring and adductor magnus stretching. This may both reduce mucus production in the way we have described for other inverted postures and calm the tense, reactive response that most people have to a stuffy nose. Put metaphorically, this pose resets the body's thermostat for tension, irritability and, in some instances I have observed, even temperature.

Contraindications: Severe osteoporosis, acute herniated lumbar intervertebral disc, severe glaucoma, colostomy, torn Achilles tendon or tendinitis.

Helpful Hints: Distribute weight evenly on each foot. Bend from the hips, not the waist. Don't hurry through it.

The Pose: Stand with feet parallel, weight evenly distributed on your feet. René Caillet, an authority on musculoskeletal medicine, divides the weight-bearing of the feet into twelve parts: six for the heel, two for the big toe and one for each of the others. Your weight should be evenly shared between the forefoot and the heel, and inner and outer parts of each foot.

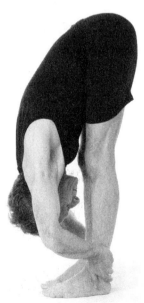

Pause for a moment to secure yourself. Raise your kneecaps firmly as you lower your palms to the floor, bending from the hips. Keep your neck somewhat extended.

Breathe quietly for a minute or two, pressing the front of your torso against your thighs, starting with your lower belly. Draw your hips forward, adjusting the weight on your palms until your legs are vertical. After a minute or two, advance your palms behind your heels, or alternatively grasp your ankles and draw your torso down rather than closer to your legs. After doing so, let your forehead come close to your shins. If you hold your ankles, draw your torso downward more than toward your legs. In any event, avoid rounding your back. Breathe slowly for several minutes, sensing the pressure of your abdomen and chest against your legs. Finish by walking your hands up your shins to your knees, then bend your knees slightly as you stand up.

LESS CHALLENGING VARIATION:
If you cannot reach the floor, use a chair or a block; go as far as you can safely.

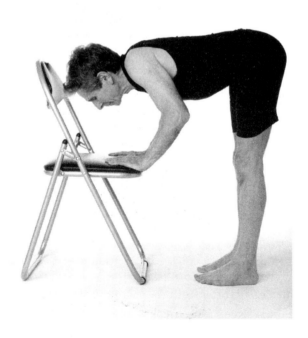

Virabhadrasana II
Warrior II Pose

Benefits and How It Works: Effectively opposes stiffness in joints and muscles of both upper and lower extremities, trunk and neck. There is no clear evidence about how this pose might reduce the symptoms of a common cold; possibly it is just the extreme exertion involved in sustaining the posture for a full minute that works, the way "sweating it out" can do away with a stuffy nose by resetting the body's homeostatic parameters.

Contraindications: Plantar fasciitis, severe internal derangement of the knee such as meniscal tears in posterior horns, advanced chondromalacia patellae, end-stage arthritis, congestive heart failure, extreme weakness or imbalance, rotator cuff syndrome.

Helpful Hints: Use a sticky mat to minimize slipping. Arch your back as little as possible. Keep your hands level, as if they were the arms of a balance scale. Maintain as vertical a torso as possible.

The Pose: Stand with your weight evenly distributed between your feet and across each foot: toes to heel, inner side to outer. Use the formula that

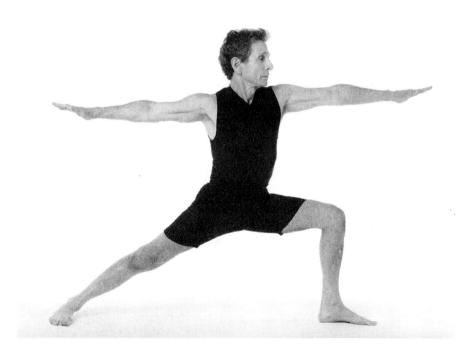

divides the weight on each foot into twelve equal parts: allot two parts to the big toe and its part of the ball of the foot, one to each smaller toe, and six to the heel of each foot. Step or spring your feet four to four and a half feet apart. Turn your left foot out 90 degrees, parallel to the side of your mat, and your right foot in 30 degrees. Bring your arms out to the sides, palms down. Keeping your torso vertical—let it descend rather than inclining toward either leg—bend your left knee until it makes a 90-degree angle. Both arms and both legs should be in one plane. Reestablish the distribution of weight on your feet. Press the big toe of your right foot into the mat while revolving the right hip and knee upward and outward to ground the outer edge of the foot. Straighten the spine from head to sacrum. Gaze along your left arm just past your middle finger.

Breathe normally and evenly for one minute. Rise up to the spread leg position and repeat the pose on the right side, after turning the left foot out 90 degrees and the right foot in 30 degrees. Come up after one minute on the right side, turn the feet parallel and jump your legs together.

VARIATIONS:

1. You can do the pose with a block under the front foot. This will tend to bend the knee a little further, unless you rock the weight backward onto the straight leg, protecting the front knee. See page 65 for an example.
2. Support your pelvis on a chair. Then gradually raise yourself off the chair to increase the energy you put into the pose. Hold it to make it as challenging as you like. See page 64 for an example with Warrior I.

If Warrior II by itself doesn't help, you should practice the entire Warrior trilogy. See pages 63 and 131. Also try other arduous standing poses such as Parivrtta Parsvakonasana (p. 81) and Parsvottanasana (p. 67).

Modified Savasana
Corpse Pose

Benefits and How it Works: Restful.

Contraindications: Late pregnancy (do the pose lying on your side).

The Pose: Sometimes a cold is so severe that you will need to modify the pose in order to avoid aggravating your symptoms. Set yourself up for a restorative Corpse Pose by placing a bolster over a stair-step arrangement of two blocks, so that the bolster is on an incline. Then you can lie face up with the pelvis on the floor and your head at the upper end of the incline. This is especially helpful if you start coughing when you lie flat. The legs can be straight, or you can support your knees with a rolled-up blanket. Alternatively, your legs can be spread apart so the soles of the feet face each other and make firm contact. Your knees should float downward or be supported by blocks.

All these poses may vanquish the cold—make it go away before your yoga session ends. Sometimes, however, yoga will just diminish the cold's symptoms and hasten the end of it.

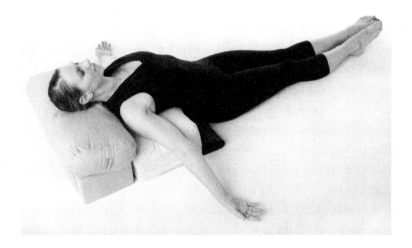

CHAPTER THIRTEEN

Bone Health

I N THE LATE 1890s, the invention of X-rays made bones inside a living body visible for the first time. Until then there was no way to assess whether a person had weak or brittle bones unless he or she was prone to fractures. Today we know that osteoporosis affects a huge percentage of the population. But while X-rays were a great innovation in that they could identify a fracture, they provided only a qualitative idea when it came to bone mineral density. There were no numbers, no benchmarks, for diagnosing the amount of bone loss that results from bodily changes, inactivity, and aging.

The better part of a century elapsed before a medical physicist named John Cameron invented bone densitometry in the 1960s, using a tiny amount of radiation to determine the exact quantity of mineral content in human bone.[1] One of this intelligent and resourceful man's early discoveries was the change in bone mineral density of lactating mothers. His research led directly to the development of the DEXA scan, the tool now used to measure bone density accurately and to diagnose osteopenia (low bone mineral density in those at risk for developing osteoporosis) and the slow progression of osteopenia that leads to full-blown osteoporosis.

The DEXA scan has opened the door for a great deal of scientific research into the disease we call osteoporosis. There is statistical information: as many as half of all women and a quarter of men older than fifty will risk a fracture due to osteoporosis.[2] That's hundreds of millions of people worldwide. Osteoporosis causes more than 8.9 million fractures a year, according to the International Osteoporosis Foundation, which means one osteoporotic fracture every three seconds! Some of these fractures are life-threatening. And yet this disease is often called silent, because people who have it are rarely aware of it until they break a bone or have a DEXA scan.

Osteoporosis, the weakening and thinning of the bones, does not take place with complete consistency. That's part of the reason that some osteoporotic fractures—spine, wrist and femur—are more common than others. Still, the disease is systemic and advances as time passes, eventually affecting all the bones in a person's body.

Without going into all the technical details of the DEXA scan, the bottom line is that the lower the bone mineral density as measured by the DEXA scan, the higher the risk of fracture. An excellent study of nearly 200,000 postmenopausal American females of five ethnicities showed that for each decrease of one standard deviation in bone mineral density (BMD) below the mean set by the 25- to 30-year-old women, there is a 50 percent increase in the risk of fracture.[3]

Your DEXA Scan

A DEXA scan is usually done on lumbar vertebrae, the hip and the top of the thighbone. It's a short, painless procedure, something like an X-ray. The result comes to you in two measurements, each comparing you to different normals: the average BMD of healthy 25- to 30-year-old women, and the average BMD of people your age.

T Score: The T score is the more important measure. It tells you how your bone mineral density compares to that of a large cohort of healthy 25- to 30-year-old women, whose bones are at the peak of their strength. Your score is measured by standard deviations—how far away you are from normal in terms of what percentage of people deviate that far. As I said above, one standard deviation below the mean (weighted average) tells you that you are 50 percent more likely to have a fracture than if you were right at the mean of these 25- to 30-year-old women. Osteopenia is defined as one standard deviation below the mean. If you have that score, it's time to worry a little about your bones. More than 2.5 standard deviations below the mean tells you that that your bones are weaker than 99 percent of the 25- to 30-year-old healthy women. That's osteoporosis. Each standard deviation you go below the mean involves another 50 percent rise in your likelihood of having a fracture. If your T score is 3.5 standard deviations below the mean, you're 50 percent more likely to have a fracture than you were at 2.5 standard deviations below.

So, summing up: how do you read your T score? A T score of −2.5 or lower tells you and your physician that you have osteoporosis. A T score of −1.0 to −2.5 indicates lower than normal bone density, which is interpreted as osteopenia.

Z Score: The Z score compares you to people of your own age and gender. So if you are 80 years old, your bone density is compared with other 80-year-olds of your gender. Therefore, as you get older, your Z score may stay the same. But your T score—your comparison with people 25 to 30 years old—is likely to go down.

Even as your age advances, you can still add bone through medication, supplements and exercise. I believe yoga is particularly beneficial, and I outline the reasons below.

Risk Factors

If you're older and female, you have a greater risk of losing bone. People who have osteoporosis in their families, who are small, Caucasian or Asian, who have diets poor in calcium and magnesium or who have low hormone levels or thyroid or parathyroid problems or chronically use steroids are at higher risk. A sedentary lifestyle can lead a person straight to osteoporosis, and while I believe wholeheartedly in yoga to arrest and reverse it, any vigorous exercise—walking, running, jumping, dancing, weightlifting—helps. African Americans have the strongest bones; Europeans are second, Asians third. Yet Asians have the lowest rate of fracture. Maybe it's because they put a higher value on good balance and therefore have fewer falls; in some cases, they are closer to the ground.[4]

Most but certainly not all of my patients who have osteoporosis are women, and many are worried that suddenly their bones are going to collapse. They feel frail and they're afraid of the drugs, most of which have deservedly bad reputations. These women don't know what to do. Taking calcium and vitamin D, which many of them have done for some time, hasn't done much good. They're afraid to hurt themselves with vigorous exercise, possibly breaking the bones they are striving to protect.

My patients influenced my decision to start a clinical trial to study the effects of yoga on osteoporosis. Not only was I interested (and optimistic), I also wanted to add to the growing body of scientific research on the efficacy of yoga for conditions ranging from back pain (Karen Sherman) to carpal tunnel syndrome (Miriam Garfinkle) to neurological problems (Shirley Telles) and diabetes (Kim Innes). A little later, I'll go into detail about my clinical trial studying yoga for osteoporosis. Who would have thought a condition unidentified until sixty years ago would be treated by the ancient practice of yoga?

Why Use Yoga for Osteoporosis

Several factors suggested it would be worthwhile to start a clinical trial to see if yoga could influence bone density.

Weight-bearing: Interesting research is being done at the University of California, where Dr. Gail Greendale, George Salem and others are using computer mapping on patients while they do yoga. This is an ingenious way to find the exact places where stresses and activations occur in muscles and joints.[5] In a simple Tree Pose, for instance, even when the pose is done only partially, with the bent leg supported on the ankle of the straight leg, bone-building stress is placed on the straight leg. So it's not just the weight-bearing of Downward Dog on a person's arms and legs; it's also the almost inevitable shifting from one side to the other and concentration of forces in balancing poses that enhances the gravitational forces and those generated in the person's own body.

Pressure: Much yoga is a study in isometrics—static exercise, where muscle length and joint angles don't change and limbs don't go through any range of motion, but tension is exerted by the muscle. Most forward bends have hamstrings and gluteus muscles opposed by quadriceps and arm muscles. That strengthens the femur (thigh bone), the tibia (shin bone), the fibula (calf bone) and the many bones of the foot. Because forward bends form a loop linking hands and feet, every bone in between is stimulated. It also puts pressure on the spine, pelvis, shoulder and arm bones. Forward and back bends globally strengthen because muscle forces are communicated everywhere from shoulders to feet. But folks who already have low BMD are limited.

Balance and Posture: No matter how weak your bones are, you are not likely to fracture one unless you slouch, fall or are on a medicine that causes a spontaneous fracture. Many studies show that yoga improves balance and posture, including one done at the University of Indiana with people who had chronic stroke.[6] Balance and lower limb strength are, of course, critical elements in avoiding falls. Many asana such as Parivrtta Ardha Chandrasana (Revolved Half Moon Pose, p. 93) and Vasisthasana (Side Plank Pose, p. 182) improve balance. Whatever else it does, yoga stretches joint capsules as well as muscles, both of which tend to contract with advancing age and reduced activity. Yoga produces better range of motion so you can more effectively extend your legs or arms to keep yourself erect when balance is disturbed, and stop yourself from falling. Obviously, all this increases your ability to right yourself if you're about to fall.[7]

Yoga also increases confidence and physical coordination and lessens anxiety—all of which improve posture and prevent falls.

Medicines[8]

Bisphosphonates are the most popular medicines for bone loss, and in my opinion, the worst. There are a lot of them, and they have a poor track record when it comes to side effects, especially with long-term use: "Data on safety have raised concern regarding the optimal duration of use for achieving and maintaining protection against fractures," according to an article in the *New England Journal of Medicine*.[9] "Further investigation into the benefits and risks of long-term therapy, as well as surveillance of fracture risk after discontinuation of bisphosphonate therapy, will be crucial for determining the best regimen of treatment for individual patients with osteoporosis," the article concludes. Drugs such as Fosomax and Boniva are taken to build bone, yet the side effects include slow healing of fractures, death of some bone tissue and spontaneous fractures in the very people who are taking these drugs to avoid breaking bones!

To appreciate how bone mineral density is gained or lost, it's necessary to understand the function of two types of cells: osteocytes, which create the protein substance that attracts calcium and phosphorus to make bone, and osteoclasts, which dissolve bone, returning the protein and minerals to the systemic circulation. Control over the number of each type of cell and their activity is complex, influenced by nutrition, medicines, hormones, body metabolism and genetic factors currently under study. We do know specifically that osteocytes are stimulated to produce bone by pressure on them.

Wolf's Law, first articulated over a century ago, states that the architectonic of any bone follows the lines of force to which the bone is exposed. By a process known as mechanotransduction, sufficient pressure against the osteoblasts' cell membrane up-regulates certain DNA and down-regulates other DNA, transforming the cell into a good osteocyte. Consistent pressure over time will stimulate enough new bone production to strengthen the femur, for example, enough so that further pressure does not deform the bone, and does not stimulate the osteocytes. This feedback mechanism sensitively governs when bone production starts and stops. It will begin again if the pressure grows or the bone weakens. In the meantime the osteocytes change their function back to preserving the well-being of the bone they have already laid down. They form long "conga lines" of cells to transport oxygen, glucose and proteins from an often distant blood vessel to the cells in the interior of every bone.

Osteoclasts are astonishingly powerful dissolvers of the bones that otherwise last thousands of years in catacombs and cemeteries. Using potent acids and enzymes, these fifty-nucleus mega-cells are called upon to dissolve bone that is unhealthy and then to signal osteocytes to get working to replace it. Together with the osteocytes, the osteoclasts' function completes the give-and-take, the constant metabolism of live bone, every molecule of which is replaced every seven years.

The bisphosphonates such as Fosamax, Boniva and Zomax (the most popular anti-osteoporosis medications at this writing), as well as newer medicines such as denosumab, work by decreasing the activity of the osteoclasts; the bone-making osteocytes are allegedly unaffected. Under the influence of these medicines, the same amount of bone is created while less bone is dissolved. That means a net gain in bone and an improved DEXA score. But when the osteoclasts are inhibited from their janitorial work of clearing away dead and diseased regions of bone, the healthy bone further from a blood vessel—further out along the conga line—does not get essential nutrients, and more and more bone gets progressively distressed. This may account for the increased osteonecrosis (bone death), hundreds of spontaneous fractures and slow healing after fractures that are seen in people taking these medicines.

In case the information above isn't enough to encourage you to do yoga, I will add that oral bisphosphonates are hard on the stomach and may be associated with other problems such as atrial fibrillation.[10] The newer intravenous versions bypass the stomach, but they are associated with scleritis, episcleritis, uvitis and other conditions of the eyes as well as the inhibition of osteoclast activity noted above.

A final word: once you take these medications, they remain in your bones forever. Other osteoporosis medicines are associated with pulmonary embolism, blood clots and stroke. Compare these charming side effects with the side effects of yoga: improved balance, greater strength, expanded range of motion, better posture, enhanced coordination and lower anxiety—all of which mitigate the risk of falling.

Supplements

A HEALTHY DIET, CALCIUM AND VITAMIN D

I believe that everyone should eat a calcium-rich diet—green leafy vegetables such as spinach and kale, dairy products, soy, sardines and salmon. These foods build strong bones in the young and help maintain them as we grow older. By the same token, a poor diet—too many colas and/or alcoholic beverages, smoking tobacco—has a negative impact on bone health. A study in the Endocrine Society's *Journal of Clinical Endocrinology and Metabolism* showed that two years of following a Mediterranean diet enriched with olive oil is associated with increased serum osteocalcin concentrations, suggesting a protective effect on bone.[11]

For many years the conventional wisdom has been that women, especially those who have reached menopause, need calcium and vitamin D supplements to help prevent fractures. I am in favor of that supplementation. Nevertheless, a dramatic study is creating controversy by suggesting that extra calcium and vitamin D might not be necessary.

"Vitamin D and calcium are part of a healthy diet. Most people can achieve sufficient doses with a healthy diet," says Dr. Kirsten Bibbins-Domingo, an associate professor of medicine at the University of California, San Francisco, who was part of the task force that looked at 137 studies of the effectiveness of vitamin D and calcium supplements. According to the task force, which did *not* say people who have osteoporosis should stop taking calcium and vitamin D, too much of these substances may lead to kidney stones in a small number of women.[12] Other studies associate calcium supplements with cardiac arrhythmias in people over the age of seventy-five. I recommend only 500 milligrams daily after that age.

METALLICS AND OTHER SUBSTANCES

Recommending specific amounts of the metallics thought to be beneficial for bone health is a tricky business, according to a review article in *Open Orthopaedics Journal*. "Some essential nutrients for bone health are readily available in the typical American diet. These include zinc, manganese and copper," say the authors. "These nutrients are usually consumed in amounts that meet or exceed the recommended dietary allowance, so they should not need supplementation unless a disease state is present. Regardless of wide availability, these metals are frequently added to dietary supplements. It should be noted that high levels of supplementation with zinc, manganese and copper may have deleterious effects."

It may be appropriate to take supplements of calcium, vitamin D, magnesium, silicon, vitamin K and boron, according to the paper. However, most people don't need extra zinc, manganese, copper and other metals, and too much of these substances can be harmful. Though there has been quite a bit of research suggesting that strontium is helpful for osteoporosis, the authors here believe more study is necessary. They do also recommend small amounts of zinc for vegetarians.[13]

More research is being done on all of this, and I look forward to seeing the results. In the meantime, we appear to have found something nontoxic that works.

My Clinical Trial for Osteoporosis

As long ago as my thirties, when I was in India studying with Mr. Iyengar, I thought about yoga and bones. Looking at him, his guru (who was said to be well over one hundred years old) and other yogis, it seemed obvious that yoga had a beneficial effect. As far as I know, Mr. Iyengar has never had a fracture, and at this writing he is in his mid-nineties. After I returned from India, I went to medical school and joined the residency program at Albert Einstein Hospital, where Dr. Edward Delagi introduced me to Julius Wolff's work.

Eventually I went into private practice, and out of curiosity and with some hope I decided to try yoga with some of my patients. I had been thinking about this for decades by that time. Over the course of a year, about 300 people did yoga with me in weekly classes. Then I asked those with osteopenia or osteoporosis if they would like to join a study. These people were losing bone—that much I knew. I didn't give them vitamin D, I didn't give them calcium. Some of them were taking supplements and some weren't. I did no tests of any kind, except a DEXA scan at the beginning and the end of the two-year test period. I knew vitamin D and calcium would do some good, but I just wanted to see if yoga worked.

During those two years, study participants came and went. Many didn't have the discipline to do yoga regularly, some moved away, some just lost interest. Still, when the two years were up, I did have some data. The problem was I didn't know exactly what my data meant. One day, when I was talking to my very intelligent, mathematically-oriented son on the phone, I said I didn't think the results of my study were statistically significant because so many people had dropped out over the two-year period. Of the original 300, only ten or twelve in the group that did yoga and eight in the control group remained. He said, "Let's see. Send me the data." He went over it all, applied SSAS (a statistical program) and got back to me about fifteen minutes later, saying, "Your results are statistically significant!" That, of course, was wonderful news. Though what I had done was a pilot study with a relatively small number of people, it strongly suggested that yoga could help people with osteoporosis arrest and reverse bone loss. I got the information together and published the results as "Yoga for Osteoporosis: A Pilot Study."[14]

It seemed that if such a small sample was statistically significant, I could make a better, more complete study—do it in a general way and with a larger number of people, and learn more. I discussed it with colleagues and came up with a plan for a small battery of blood tests and a urine test to look for bone turnover. If the patient was taking medication for bone loss, I estimated how much bone they had gained before joining the study and projected how much they would gain while taking the medication and doing yoga. I asked them to have hip-joint X-rays to measure the advance of any arthritis, and before-and-after spine films to detect fractures, but those weren't mandatory. Anyone who was willing to take the blood and urine tests and get a DEXA scan, and agreed to do the yoga, could join.

Since I was asking for study participants through my website and expected to have far-flung participants whom I had never met, I made a DVD so that everyone would be doing virtually the same thing for the same length of time. Everyone would have the same "dose." I thought about poses very carefully, avoided forward bends that are known to cause fracture, and included a lot of poses that work the hips and lower back because they are measured on the DEXA scan. I emphasized back bends and twists. This was kind of gutsy, because much of the yoga community believed then, and still does, that twists are bad for osteoporosis. Even the National Osteoporosis Foundation advises against twists.[15] But in more than 70,000 hours of my study, with people doing three twists daily following the way they are done in my instructional video, there has been no report or X-ray, indicating a new fracture related to yoga.

At this writing, more than seven years from the beginning of the pilot study and five years after the beginning of the bigger study with the DVD, my trials have involved 800 participants from all over North America and five other continents. People still drop out because they can't stick with the daily twelve-minute yoga routine, but again I have results. So far forty-four patients—all of them losing bone when they started the yoga—have reported their two-year follow-up. Of these forty-four, thirty-six are *gaining* bone two years later. That's about 82 percent. Obviously, more study is needed. Still, I cannot help but be hopeful about the inexpensive, portable tool of yoga for the hundreds of millions who suffer from bone loss.

I am also studying bone quality, the cutting edge in evaluating bone's resistance to fracture. Bone quality includes the bone mineral density measured by the DEXA scan, but adds a computational analysis of how well the supports within the bone are oriented and combined. In a manner similar to the way engineers calculate the strength of a bridge or an airplane wing, finite element analysis is being used at New York University and the University of Pennsylvania to examine our study patients' bones. The study is going on now, and the information we have now suggests that compared to other people in the study, yogis have better bone quality.

Preventive Yoga for Those with Weak Bones

The work I've done on maintaining healthy bone mineral density has been directed at people who are already at risk or who have osteoporosis. All the poses presented below are cautiously designed to put pressure on fragile bones. However, the most useful application of yoga might be for prevention.

When it comes to prevention—starting with normal bones and doing what we can to keep them healthy—we would use entirely different poses, which bring much greater, but still tolerable pressures to bear. I recommend intense forward bends for these healthy young people, and we would get as close as possible to Dwi Pada Sirsasana (Ankles Behind the Neck Pose) as the pose of choice. This is an advanced and difficult pose; any that approach it in the pressures on the fronts of the vertebrae are highly recommended. People under thirty are building bone and will benefit from putting substantial pressure on their bones. A vigorous and challenging regimen is appropriate for yoga practiced in schools and colleges, as students' bones are optimally responsive. For more, see Fishman and Saltonstall, *Yoga for Osteoporosis.*

I have included below one pose meant to strengthen the anterior vertebral bodies, where fractures commonly take place. Strengthening the anterior part of the vertebrae in people whose bones are weak is a delicate matter. Direct force such as that produced by forward bends has been shown to raise the risk of fracture, so they are out of the question. Twists apply moderate radial forces and stimulation to the osteocytes of the vertebral bodies. In spite of the controversy, I have seen no adverse effects on X-rays or elsewhere in my study participants who have done so many thousands of hours of yoga with twists. Recent cadaveric studies support this notion.[16]

Osteoporosis makes every bone in the body liable to fracture. In our studies we have focused on the spine, hip and thigh bone, both because they are the most frequently fractured and because most of the studies in osteoporosis measure the bone mineral density at those sites. The wrists, ribs and feet are also at sizable risk. The poses below put bone-building pressures on many of these bones, without any trauma to the joints that I know of.

Vrksasana
Tree Pose

Benefits and How It Works: Safely challenges and gradually improves balance. Applies vertical and lateral pressure to the hip and spine that stimulates osteocytes and strengthens bones. Enhances alertness, focus and symmetry.

Contraindications: Severe balance issues, severe rotator cuff syndrome, plantar fasciitis or shoulder impingement, ankle instability while standing.

Helpful Hints: Distribute your weight evenly and firmly on the standing foot; look intently at a point level with your eyes; expand your side ribs as you raise your arms overhead, stretching them upward as far as possible.

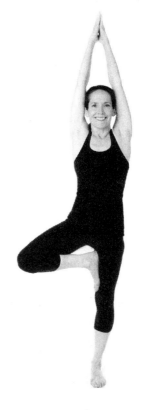

The Pose: Stand with your feet together, toes spread out. Press your left foot firmly into the floor. Consciously, but moderately, tighten the left quadriceps and hamstrings, making the whole thigh firm. Open your hip joints by tucking the bottom of your pelvis forward. This should reduce your lumbar curve. Align your pelvis directly above your feet. Raise your right foot to the top of your left thigh, toes pointing toward the left ankle. Keep the pelvis facing forward as you open the right thigh out to the side (ideally at 90 degrees to the left foot). Reopen the hips by tucking the lower pelvis forward. Refocus your gaze at a point at eye level, 15–20 feet away. Slowly inhale as you raise your arms symmetrically, turning the palms inward to meet above your head. Let your lungs fill completely.

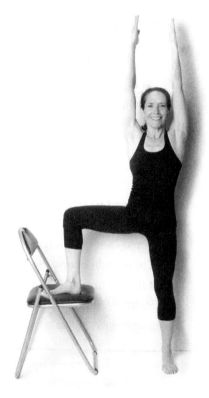

Holding your shoulders back, stretch up from your left ankle to your fingertips. Stretch upward, trying to leave only the skin of the sole of your foot fixed to the earth. Take a few calm, normal breaths. Let your arms descend as you exhale. Slowly repeat the cycle of arm elevation and breathing several times. Come out of the pose slowly, placing both feet squarely on the floor. Repeat, reversing legs.

LESS CHALLENGING VARIATIONS:

1. Place the side of a chair against a wall so it faces you. Stand to the right of the chair with your back against the wall. Place your right foot on the seat of the chair, then proceed as above. This version does nothing to strengthen your bones beyond what normal weight-bearing would do, but it is a sensible way to start challenging your balance.

2. Do the pose against the wall but without a chair. As long as your right foot rests on the left leg, the forces that are brought to bear on the right hip are at least 60 percent greater than gravity alone.

Salabhasana
Locust Pose

Benefits and How It Works: Puts bone-building pressure on facet joints behind the vertebral bodies and on the pelvis. Safely and quickly builds strength in the posterior parts of the spine. Suitable for those with wrist weakness.

Contraindications: Abdominal hernias, -ostomies, severe spinal stenosis.

Helpful Hints: Soften the abdominal muscles or they will inhibit the extension inherent in the pose. Draw the back of your head back from your throat to lengthen your spine; do not just tip your head upward. Increase lift by bringing your shoulders back, together, and toward your pelvic rim as you inhale.

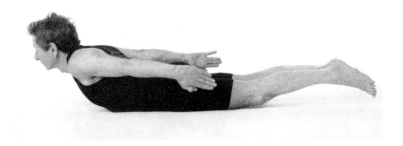

The Pose: Lie prone with your arms straight out behind you and your fingers interlaced behind your back. Elongate your body from head to toe and puff out your chest to increase your vertebral range of motion. Slowly and carefully raise your shoulders, followed by your trunk, then your neck and head. Focus on lifting your throat rather than your head.

Slide your hands down toward your thighs as you raise your straight legs off the floor. Retract your shoulders and elongate your arms behind you as far as possible. Engage your back muscles to lift both your torso and your thighs. Relax your belly. Tight abdominal muscles will prevent your back from arching as we want it to. Come down by lowering your legs first, then bring your hands underneath your shoulders and lower the chest, neck and head.

VARIATIONS:

1. Begin with your hands underneath your shoulders. Follow the steps above but do not lift your legs.
2. Begin with your arms at your sides, externally rotating your shoulders to turn your palms outward.
3. Begin with your arms at your sides, palms facing your thighs.

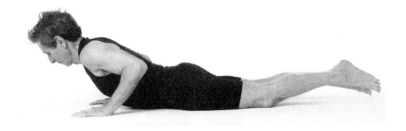

4. To strengthen your back extensors even more quickly, begin with your arms stretched out horizontally in front of you.

5. To improve scapular stabilization, an important element in balance, hold your arms out horizontally to either side, airplane style.

6. Grasp just above the ankles of the yoga friend who is straddling your prone frame, just about at hip level. The friend then places the palm of a straightened right arm on your spine at T4 (fourth thoracic vertebra). Her left fingertips gently hold your sacrum in place and steady her balance. You may pull gently on her ankles to increase your trunk and leg's

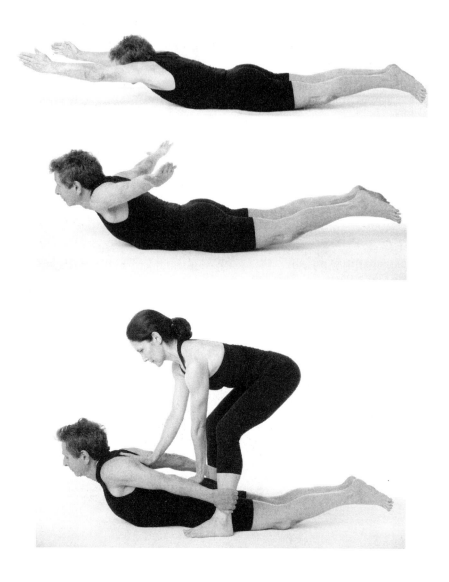

elevation. The friend may also tiptoe back and then slowly descend onto her heels. In the latter case, your elbows should be straight before she descends.

Parivrtta Parsvakonasana
Revolved Side Angle Pose

Benefits and How It Works: This pose generates sufficient force to strengthen almost every bone in the body. It promotes agility, which improves coordination, and has a challenging balance component. This arduous pose also develops endurance, which reduces your risk of falling when you're fatigued.

Contraindications: Repeated shoulder subluxation, Hill–Sachs deformity, Bankart lesion, total hip replacement, intervertebral disc herniation, grade II or more severe spondylolisthesis, balance issues, anterior cruciate ligament injury, chondromalacia patellae, Dupuytrens contracture, carpal tunnel syndrome. In rotatory scoliosis, do the pose only to the side opposite the bulge. (In right buldge, bend the left knee.)

Helpful Hints: Place your hand squarely on the floor to maintain balance, and proceed carefully. Elongate your whole body, toes to fingertips. Breathe into both sides of your chest.

The Pose: Kneel facing the long way on a yoga mat. Raise your left thigh, placing your left foot straight ahead, far enough in front of you to make a right angle behind the left knee. Gently twist to bring your right chest and

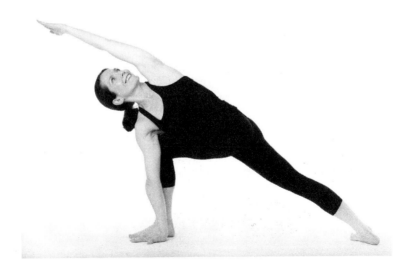

shoulder over the left thigh and extend your right arm on the outside of the left shin. Place your right palm squarely on the mat, fingers stretching forward.

Begin to press the outside of your right upper arm against the outside of the left knee as you twist your right hip forward. Pull your left shoulder backward. Rest your left hand on your left flank. Breathe slowly and symmetrically to elongate your torso.

For the full pose, straighten your right leg, taking care that the foot is angled 30 degrees inward and its fifth toe is touching the mat. Retain the 90-degree angle of the left knee and extend the left arm diagonally over your head behind your ear. Your left hand, arm, torso and leg should be in a straight line. Again, make your torso as long as possible, and breathe slowly and symmetrically.

LESS CHALLENGING VARIATIONS:

1. Place the left buttock on the edge of a chair. Stretch the left thigh in front of you, knee bent to 90 degrees, and the right behind you with the knee as straight as possible. Use your hands on the seat and back of the chair to gently revolve the right hip and torso forward.

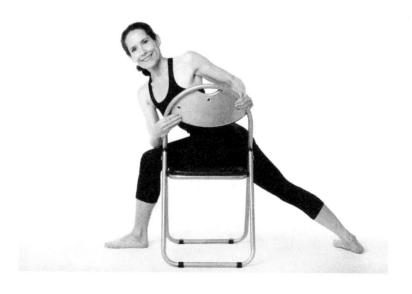

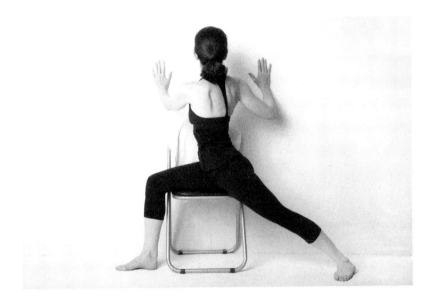

2. You may wish to do this version with the back of the chair against a wall. Your right leg should be the one closer to the wall. After you turn your left torso and shoulder forward and over the right thigh, place both palms against the wall. Use your left hand for balance, and your right to gently and carefully twist your entire torso. Then reverse, using the left thigh.

Viranchyasana
Ankles Behind Neck Pose

This pose is for *prevention* of osteoporosis and osteopenia, and is *only* to be done by healthy people with reasonably strong bones. In people with weakened bones, the pressures it exerts may cause fractures. For healthy people, forward bends such as Janusirsasana (p. 34) and Krounchasana (p. 224) lead up to this pose. These, too, should be performed only by those without osteopenia or osteoporosis or other bone conditions such as osteogenesis imperfect.

Benefits and How It Works: Builds strong vertebral bodies by exerting pressure on their anterior regions. The posture stimulates osteocytes to deposit more protein, leading to more and stronger bone. The inner architecture of the bone may be affected as well, as research should make clear within the next few years.

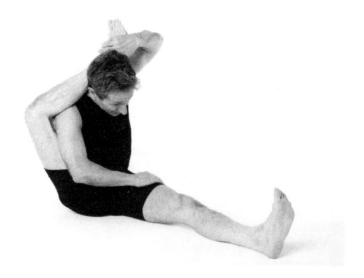

Contraindications: Osteopenia, osteoporosis, compression fracture, herniated disc, severe hip arthritis, tight hamstrings.

The Pose: Sit on the floor, legs extended. Exhale. Grasp your right leg just below the knee, raising it toward the lower chin. Take a breath. Cradle the right ankle with the left hand and exhale as you raise the right calf above your head and into the crook of the back of your neck. Straighten your back gently but firmly, looking up until your gaze is close to true horizontal. Take several breaths as normally as possible. Inhale as you release the right leg. Take a few slow breaths before repeating the pose on the left side.

This pose leads up to Dwi Pada Sirsasana, in which both legs rest behind the neck simultaneously.

CHAPTER FOURTEEN

Insomnia

THE PURPOSE OF sleep isn't completely understood, but we do know that it's important for heart health, for learning and memory, for healing, even for life. Studies done on rats have shown that if they are deprived of REM (rapid eye movement sleep, which is normal for long periods every night), their life cycle is shortened almost by half. How long a person needs to sleep depends on the individual, but everyone needs more or less sleep at different stages of life. Infants, for example, sleep as much as eighteen hours a day, adolescents about ten hours, and most normal adults need seven or eight hours. Some adults, though they know sleep is important, go to bed late and get up early, choosing not to get their optimal amount of rest, which eventually takes a toll. As people get older their pattern of sleep changes, as does the time they spend in REM sleep: older people tend to wake more times during the night, decreasing the amount of REM sleep they get. This sometimes makes them feel they aren't sleeping well or aren't sleeping enough.[1]

Recent work by Maiken Ledergaard suggests that in the third level of sleep, just before we enter REM sleep, the central nervous system is suffused with lymph-like fluid which washes out toxins and other products of its metabolism. Since the brain and spinal cord have no lymphatic system whatever, sleep would seem to produce a phenomenon that irrigates the central nervous system much the way the tides cleanse the seashore.

Insomnia—difficulty in falling asleep, or inability to fall asleep or to stay asleep for as long as you want, or to sleep restfully—plagues nearly everyone from time to time. According to the National Lung, Blood and Heart Institute, a third of adults experience occasional insomnia, and one-tenth of the adult population lives with chronic insomnia. This makes one feel tired and out of sorts during the day and is associated with absenteeism, accidents and depression.[2] A French study found that insomnia caused difficulty with memory and paying attention, led to increased anxiety and of course made people sleepy. Insomnia had a particularly negative effect on those who took antidepressants, causing more troubles during the day.[3]

Clearly, insomnia is something to avoid. If you have it, you must deal with it effectively. I'm lucky because I can usually fall asleep in a few seconds, even when lying on the floor, and I am a champion napper, which reinvigorates me and helps when I don't sleep enough at night. Sometimes, if I am thinking about a project, trying to solve a problem or worrying about someone or something, I wake up at 4 am. If I can't go back to sleep, I'm doomed to feel tired and function poorly the next day—unless I do yoga that I've devised to do right then and there, in bed in the middle of the night. Sometimes I get up and creep to a quiet place in the living room to prepare myself to sleep again, and to sleep well. Yoga works for me 99 percent of the time.

My wife says the fear of not being able to fall asleep can actually become a self-fulfilling prophecy, keeping her from falling asleep or from going back to sleep if she wakes up during the night. For her, even being overtired after a busy day makes it difficult to wind down enough to get the proper shuteye.

Insomnia is an immensely complex phenomenon. It can last a few days or a week, or it can be chronic; it can drive you to your wits' end. Difficulty falling asleep or staying asleep may be primary—that is, the insomnia may not have a discoverable cause. But sleeplessness is also associated with many other disorders: anxiety and depression are two major ones. It can be caused by sleep apnea (abnormal pauses in breathing during sleep), restless legs syndrome or just aging.[4] Travel to different time zones can cause insomnia, as can aches and pains, heartburn, medications taken for various illnesses, the illnesses themselves, a sedentary way of life and obesity. "Evidence is growing that sleep is a powerful regulator of appetite, energy use, and weight control," according to "Your Guide to Healthy Sleep," published by the National Institutes of Health.[5]

Unfortunately, millions of Americans try to solve their sleep problems with over-the-counter and prescription drugs.[6] Many of these substances have a long half-life, which can cause hangovers. Some are addictive. An allergic reaction to a sleep medication can be serious, and some sleep medications cause strange behaviors. Here's one example: a Nobel Prize-winner we know went to his computer after taking an Ambien because he was jet-lagged and trying to get back on schedule. He wrote for hours, churning out a great many words and printing them. In the morning, he found that all he had written was gibberish.

There is a lot you can do to help yourself go to sleep and stay asleep without drugs. No heavy work late in the day. Don't drink alcoholic beverages right before bedtime. Eat dinner relatively early. Take a warm bath. Be sure your sleep environment is conducive to rest by limiting computer, television, telephone and other distractions in the bedroom. People sleep better when the room is cool rather than very warm, and of course when the bed is clean and comfortable.

Research has shown that yoga and other alternative therapies such as relaxation, tai chi and music are helpful with insomnia, whatever its cause. Of course, the cause must always be taken into consideration. In a Brazilian study, some participants who took prescription sleep medications and were dependent on them were able, after doing yoga, to reduce their dependence.[7]

The beauty of yoga for insomnia is that it kills several birds with one stone. Not only does it help young and old get more and better sleep, it also improves mood, reduces stress and ameliorates many conditions that underlie insomnia, including restless legs syndrome and osteoarthritis. A pilot study of gentle yoga for sleep disturbance in women with osteoarthritis supported the feasibility and acceptability of a standardized evening yoga practice for middle-aged to older women with osteoarthritis, and suggested that such a program would help.[8]

Another study, with seventy-five female participants, randomized and controlled, showed that the women in the yoga group had significantly greater improvement than those in the control group when it came to sleep quality and mood. They also experienced less prevalent insomnia, anxiety and perceived stress, and had lower blood pressure.[9] Yet another study done in Brazil with three groups of forty-four postmenopausal women—one group doing no exercise at all, the second doing passive stretching and the third doing yoga—showed significant benefits for the yoga group, who experienced a reduction in insomnia and menopausal symptoms, and reported better quality of life and ability to withstand stress.

To sum up, yoga provides rapid access to sleep, which "knits up the raveled sleeve of care," without cost. It yields priceless hours of sleep and an awakening without the aftermath of sedatives, hypnotics, anxiolytics or any medicines at all. Given the vast array and various functions of the billions of neurons in our central nervous system, it is critical to enter into the restful hours of slumber in a coordinated way. It may seem paradoxical that yoga can do two things simultaneously—relax you and refine your ability to coordinate sleep—but that's what it looks like when patients report after they try the following regimen.

There are three parts to this method, which has helped many patients and which I use myself. It takes a total of about seven minutes. The entire series can be done in bed. It is just as effective for going to sleep at the beginning of the night as for getting back to sleep if you awake prematurely. Many fall asleep before finishing this short routine.

Supta Padangusthasana I
Reclining Hand to Big Toe Pose

Benefits and How It Works: By stretching the golgi tendon organs within the hamstrings' tendons, these muscles are induced to relax. The pose brings a sense of floating to the legs and definitely signals "relax" to the entire central nervous system.

Contraindications: Severe hip arthritis, late pregnancy, hamstring tear.

Helpful Hints: This pose can be done in bed. Keep both knees and your back as straight as possible, and the bottom leg under the covers, against the mattress. Remove the pillow. Use a belt or towel as a prop if needed.

The Pose: Lie on your back. Lengthen your entire body, stretching your heels away from your hips and the back of your head away from your shoulders. Center your shoulderblades under your back ribs. Lift your right leg, knee straight, until you can hold your foot in both hands. Work your way out from your shin or thigh with your hands if necessary. Bend your knee if you can't reach your foot with your leg straight, or loop a belt or a towel around your foot. Keep the other leg squarely on the bed, shoulderblades centered and knees straight as you draw your leg toward your chest. Hold the pose, breathing slowly, for 20–30 seconds. Lower the leg and repeat on the other side.

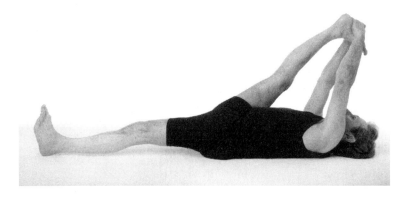

VARIATION:

Supta Padangusthasana I can also be done lying on one side. This is useful in late pregnancy. However, if you have osteoporosis or a herniated disc, be careful not to round your spine. Doing it on your side should help if you have lower back pain that gets worse when you lie on your back, but your spine will curve forward somewhat, which risks a herniated disk. If you have sleep apnea, lying on your side might be helpful.

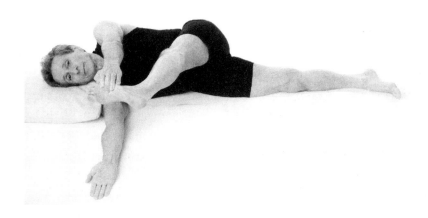

Viloma I and Viloma II
Three-Part Breath I and II

Benefits and How It Works: Slowing breathing and regulating its rhythm is at once relaxing and fatiguing. People used to this exercise become more conscious of their quiet body as other cares recede into the background.

Contraindications: Congestive heart failure, moderate or severe angina, severe sleep apnea (because one may fall asleep while practicing it).

Helpful Hints: Puff your chest up so strongly that you cannot expand much further when you inhale in Viloma I. Do not contract your chest as you exhale in Viloma II. Do not use your pillow.

The Pose: Viloma I: Lie flat on your back for sleeping, but the pose is pictured in seated position, as it is traditionally done. Close your eyes. Breathe normally for a short while until you are comfortable. Exhale. Puff up your chest before breathing in. Break up your inhalation into three smaller segments: breathe in about one-third of a breath, then stop for 2–5 seconds, breathe in a second third of a breath then stop for 2–5 seconds, then breathe

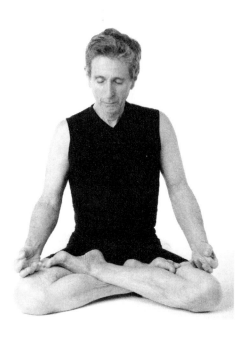

in completely. Inhale smoothly and slowly during each segment. Do not close your throat or use your tongue to stop the breathing between segments. Do not hold your breath; hold your breathing. Keep your chest large throughout the inhalation. The idea is to use your diaphragm like a piston that goes up and down in a relatively unchanging chamber. After doing Supta Padangusthasana I, you should be relaxed. Be a spectator of your process of respiration.

Do not make it a huge, exaggerated breath. It should be a normal breath, taken in slowly so it is easy to divide into three relatively equal parts. When you have completed all three thirds of the breath, pause for a moment with your lungs full before you slowly exhale. Do this all so quietly that you cannot hear yourself breathe. Then take a normal breath before inhaling in thirds again. After that take another normal breath before breathing in thirds for the third and last time.

Viloma II: Follow what you've just done in Viloma I with another normal breath. Then do the reverse: take in a full breath and exhale in three equal segments. Pause for a few seconds between each one-third exhalation. Take one normal full breath between each of the three normal inhalations and three-part exhalations. Again, keep your chest large and as motionless as possible as you exhale, and do not use your throat or tongue to retain air or stop the exhalation. Do it from the diaphragm.

If the breathing part of this anti-insomnia work is very difficult, or if you are unsure whether you are doing it correctly, a good yoga teacher will be helpful. Done carefully, with respect for your body and your capacity for rest, it should be harmless.

The third part of this sequence comes from Tantric yoga.[10] As you lie there, contemplate these ten concepts, spending approximately 30 seconds on each one. Do not time yourself. Just focus on the concept and watch your attention fade for 30 seconds or so, then take up the next one. At first you may need to have a list of the concepts by your bed, but very quickly you will know them by heart. They are:

Love
Radiance
Unity
Health
Strength
Abundance
Wisdom
Light-as-air
Inner space
Trust

Then just lie there for a few minutes. If necessary, repeat the whole procedure. Often people fall asleep before finishing the set of three activities.

I know of no series that approaches this one for promoting sleep, but there is an alternative that works most of the time: get up and do 20–30 minutes of yoga, ending with forward bends, and 20–30 minutes of still meditation, and then go to back to bed.

CHAPTER FIFTEEN

Scoliosis

ABNORMAL CURVATURE OF the spine is a lot more common than you might think, especially among women. Scoliosis affects 1–3 percent of the population—as many as nine million people in the United States. According to some authors, up to 35 percent of scoliosis patients have at least some back pain.[1] This is a far greater percentage than I have seen over the years. Every year, scoliosis patients make more than 600,000 visits to private physicians' offices in the United States, an estimated 30,000 children are fitted with a brace, an unstudied number have other conservative therapies and 38,000 patients undergo surgery. Scoliosis may be associated with cerebral palsy, tethered spinal cord and other conditions. Spine curvature can become disfiguring and in some cases life-threatening if it progresses so far as to impair cardiac function or breathing.

The most prevalent types of scoliosis are idiopathic, congenital, and neuromuscular scoliosis, though as the population ages degenerative scoliosis is becoming more common.[2] The great majority of people—80 percent—have the idiopathic type, for which no scientific cause has been discovered though a genetic component is suspected. Idiopathic scoliosis is usually found in young people between the ages of eleven and seventeen and diagnosed by the school nurse or physical education teacher, or during a visit to the doctor.[3] According to the American Academy of Orthopaedic Surgeons, a curve of 25 to 40 degrees is considered enough to require treatment, and if conservative treatments fails and curves progress to 50 degrees or more, surgery may be indicated.[4]

I will be discussing idiopathic scoliosis and (adult) degenerative scoliosis, the most common forms, and the treatment I have developed for them here.

Scoliosis is not always the classic sideways curve of the spine, which when healthy and normal should be straight. The scoliotic spine may look like a "C" or, if it has a compensatory curve, an "S." During a physical exam, the patient is asked to remove his or her shirt and bend forward. A curve to one side or the other may be visible. If one side of the spine is more prominent than the other, it may be due to scoliosis. Other signs are uneven hips, leg length or shoulder height. X-rays are taken to confirm the diagnosis and other underlying causes are ruled out. Standard X-rays, both front and side views, are done when the patient is standing up; these also show the curves associated with kyphosis (abnormal rounding of the upper back) and lordosis (abnormal inward curve of the lumbar spine). When kyphotic and lordotic curves are normal, they reverse themselves with movement. They need to be watched, however, when they become exaggerated and/or unchanging. Scoliosis always involves a sideways curvature of the spine and is always abnormal.[5]

Can you diagnose your own scoliosis? That can be tough to do, but usually the convex curve is on the bulging side of the spine—the side toward which the spine rotates. You cannot always tell if you have secondary curves. A simple X-ray is a very low risk and dependable answer.

Once it has been diagnosed, the question about scoliosis becomes, how big is the curve and how likely is it to progress? School-based scoliosis screening is mandated in twenty-six states and many others have voluntary screening, but few of the children who are referred to doctors through these programs end up receiving treatment. My own private research has shown that yoga can help those whose curves might progress, with hardly any cost and with relative simplicity.

John Robert Cobb (1903–67), an orthopedic surgeon, developed the method for measuring scoliosis curves that is standard today. There is general agreement that the maturity of the bones being measured can be assigned a Risser number that helps in predicting whether or not scoliosis will progress and become serious. Current treatments for those who have curves of 50 degrees or more are bracing, various physical therapy techniques, the Schroth method (more about this later), chiropractic, osteopathic manipulation and surgery. While some of these methods are more or less successful, it's safe to say they are far from being proven.[6] They are also arduous, time-consuming, obtrusive and expensive. The National Scoliosis Foundation (NSF) currently says on its website that exercise alone will not prevent a curve from increasing, but that exercise combined with brace treatment may help.[7] I disagree.

Scoliosis and Yoga

I began to figure out how to use yoga to help scoliosis patients in the 1980s, when circumstances made it possible for me to experiment. The patient who started me thinking about this was a midlevel administrator at a hospital in Connecticut. She was in her late fifties at the time, a little bird of a thing, still working in spite of a heart condition. This poor woman's scoliosis had progressed enough to compromise her breathing, and her prognosis was poor. She came to see me with her daughter, a yoga teacher. That was a fortuitous event that gave me courage to propose using yoga as a treatment, though I didn't know for sure if it could help.

I said to the woman, "I'm aiming to slow the progress of your scoliosis or even to arrest it." Luckily she was game—even heroic.

Right from the beginning I suspected that yoga could strengthen the muscles that were stretched by the curvature so that those muscles could pull away from the curve and straighten the spine. I tried many things with this woman—one exercise in which she put her arm against the wall and pushed, which I thought might activate the right muscles in her back, seemed to help for a while. I tried seven or eight poses, many of them variations of Vasisthasana (Side Plank Pose), always talking them over with the woman's yoga-teaching daughter. Then, feeling her poor twisted back with my hand as she tried Vasisthasana, I decided that I had hit upon the right pose for her. I didn't know how long she should do it, but because she was an older person with a heart condition I said, "Just do it as long as you can, but do it every day. Don't make yourself crazy."

When she started, my patient had a primary curve of 109 degrees and a secondary curve in the 60s. We decided to continue our collaborative experiment for six months. She could do the pose pretty well when she started, and she was very conscientious, doing it faithfully every day. After three months, she seemed to be holding her own. After six months, I wondered if I was kidding myself to be thinking she was making progress, so I asked her to have another X-ray. It was astonishing. The primary curve had gone from 109 degrees to 65 degrees, and the secondary curve had gone from somewhere around 60 degrees to 45 degrees. She kept doing the exercises, and she kept coming to me. After a couple of years the curves were very small.

Now she and I are old friends, and she's still my occasional patient at the age of ninety-three. The scoliosis has almost vanished. Does this suggest how long a person needs to do the yoga to stop or reverse the progression of scoliosis? I confess I don't know the answer to that yet.

Conservative Treatments: Yoga, Schroth and Bracing

I am far from the only researcher trying to find nonsurgical treatments for scoliosis. Several yogis are well known for their work with scoliosis; some of them have the condition themselves. Although I have great respect for the work of some yoga teachers who have made videos and written books on this subject, I don't always agree with their conclusions or process. Many have no scientific evidence and no rationale for the poses they recommend. Unlike some of my colleagues, I believe that the weaker side of the back must be strengthened; I am not in favor of poses that are meant to reposition people rather than making particular muscles stronger.

Then there is the German Schroth method, which asserts its success and is widely believed to be effective in preventing progression of and reducing curvature. Identifying weak muscle groups and tight muscle groups is part of the regimen, and patients are urged to do exercises for half an hour a day with the aim of "de-rotating" and elongating the spine so that it becomes straight again. Clinical research has been done on the Schroth method; however, some of the articles do not measure spinal curves by the standard Cobb method and do not use accepted criteria for controlled, randomized studies. The writings present a long list of "forbidden" yoga poses, none of which I think would help or hurt much, except Triangle Pose, which I agree may be contraindicated if practiced often over long periods of time. (One well-known yogi is in favor of using Triangle Pose; the jury is out, as none of these poses have been subjected to randomized, controlled studies.) I believe Ardha Chandrasana (Half Moon Pose), which the Schroth method bans, is helpful if done with the convex side up. I have done EMG studies that confirm this.

Bracing is the long, drawn-out process which adolescents undergo until their spines stop growing—often for years—and involves wearing a hard plastic or soft fabric brace for as long as twenty-three hours a day, or in some cases just at night.[8] The consensus is that bracing helps in a minority of cases, sometimes decreasing the degree of the curve and keeping it smaller after treatment. There are also studies, in Europe and the US, that document the terrible effect of this technique on young girls: it lowers self-esteem, distorts self-image and prompts withdrawal from regular social activities. I can confirm this in my experience with patients.[9] Despite the fact that it can be psychologically injurious, it is supported by almost every health insurance company. I know of no health professional who recommends yoga, though I think it is amazingly effective and raises confidence and self-esteem, posing no visible impediment to mobility. Just before finishing the manuscript for this book I saw a patient with scoliosis, and in our discussion I mentioned that twelve-year-olds are incarcerated in a large contraption just when their bodies are changing, their intimate impulses are gathering and their peer group becomes paramount. The woman burst into tears and said, "That's exactly how I felt."

There is not enough evidence at this writing to warrant serious consideration of physical therapy, chiropractic, massage or meditation for the treatment of scoliosis.

My Yoga Treatment for Scoliosis

The spine may be seen as a tensegrity structure—Buckminster Fuller's term to describe objects of any size that are kept together by the tension between their parts. Radio antennae and tent poles that are held up vertically by downward-pulling cables are classic examples. In my view, the human spine belongs in this group. A simplified analysis of how we stand erect involves the symmetrical downward pull of muscles.

When you look at our anatomy, there is no skyhook holding us erect. The quadratus lumborum muscles must balance the ribcage, and the paraspinal muscles must keep the spinal column straight. The abdominal muscles do the same thing front-to-back and side-to side too, as they also govern rotation.

Curve				Primary Curve		Secondary Curve		Percentage Improvement		Interval between DEXAs
Patient	Gender	Age	Side	Pre-Yoga¶	Post-Yoga¶¶	Pre-Yoga	Post-Yoga	Primary	Secondary	Months
1	F	17	RT*	18	5.4			70.00%		7
2	F	71	RT	10	7			30.00%		6
3	F	82	RT/LT**	84	62	46	37	26.19%	19.57%	3
4	F	54	LT	70	47			32.86%		4.5
5	M	65	LT	28	16			42.86%		3
6	F	85	LT/RT	120	90	120	90	25.00%	25.00%	6
7	F	66	L	76	45			40.79%		3
8	F	77	LT	60	42			30.00%		3
9	F	14	RT/LT	24	15	18	12	37.50%	33.33%	3
10	M	15	LT	43	12			72.09%		6
Mean	2 males	54.67		53.30	34.14	61.33	46.33	40.73%	25.97%	4.44
SD				34.89	27.87	52.70	39.83	17.1	7.3	1.74

*RT = right; LT = left   **complex curve Right curve primary

¶ X-ray taken before yoga treatment began

¶¶ X-ray taken after yoga treatment

"SD" = standard deviation

My belief is that the usual varieties of scoliosis, adolescent idiopathic and degenerative, are explained by asymmetry in the forces these muscles exert on the spine. The spine will bend toward the stronger side; the convex side is the weaker one. The ribs on the convex side often splay out like the spokes of a wheel, and migrate backward into the space that this expansion has created. This makes the weaker, convex side look quite large, suggesting that it is the stronger side, though the reality is the opposite. Successful treatment will equalize the muscles' pull by strengthening the muscles of that bulging area. Vasisthasana (Side Plank Pose) asymmetrically strengthens the quadratus lumborum, iliopsoas and paraspinal muscles of the convex side, reducing the curve.

I have conducted a pilot study to test this theory. Before being taught Vasisthasana, study participants were given X-rays. They were asked to do the pose *only with the convex side downward* for three to six months, and then to get another X-ray. The same radiologist read the before-and-after films. In twenty-seven patients ranging in age from thirteen to eighty-seven, the average improvement was 36 percent over a mean period of 4.4 months. To confirm the theory, I put contraction-sensing electrodes onto the relevant muscles on both sides while test subjects assumed the pose. This confirmed the asymmetrical activity in the muscles. The first ten are given in the chart.

There was one muscle pair, the iliopsoas, too deep in the body to reach with EMG electrodes during the pose. I practiced for a few months until I could hold Vasisthasana reasonably motionlessly for eight minutes—long enough to complete an MRI. The images showed strong contraction of the iliopsoas on the convex side but not on the other side. If the pose is held as long as possible, people with idiopathic scoliosis seem to be able to reduce their curves within a few months.

Infants and toddlers of both genders have the same percentages of scoliosis at age seven. However, things change. By age ten to fifteen, girls with significant curves greatly outnumber boys. Two Japanese researchers in Texas have shown definitively that males become 50 percent stronger than girls between ten and fifteen years of age. To make a long story short, this translates to a significantly greater asymmetry in females that may be relevant to the development of scoliosis. Vasisthasana (Side Plank Pose) helps to even things out. Subsequent studies will be needed, but my pilot study seems to confirm the value of Vasisthasana done once daily for as long as possible with the convex side down.[10]

Since beginning to write this book I have carefully monitored each scoliosis patient that has come to me. I now have accumulated 116. Following their progress with the extremely low-dose X-rays periodically, I have found the adolescents to have a result about 10% better than those who have degenerative scoliosis, but both groups' curves reduce by 30–40% within three to four months of practicing Vasisthasana with the convex side down. We have had to adapt the practice slightly in some cases, and have found success with other poses to reduce the S-type curves, but the method presented here is clinically verified, and a twenty-five patient study with Karen Sherman, Erik Groessl and me has been accepted for publication, (Global Adv Health Med. 2014; 3 (5)) in press.

Vasisthasana
Side Plank Pose

Benefits and How It Works: Asymmetrically strengthens muscles that draw together ribs, vertebral bodies and facet joints on the convex side of the major curve. One side's muscles work hard, the other's do not.

Contraindications (for all variations): Profound weakness, Hill–Sachs deformity, Bankart fracture, shoulder subluxation, trochanteric bursitis, lateral collateral ligamentous laxity, Dupuytren's contracture, carpal tunnel syndrome, fifth metatarsal fracture, all on the convex side.

Helpful Hints: Put your upper (concave side) arm and shoulder against a wall and keep them there. Align your head with your spine. This is an exuberant pose—don't be shy about stretching your body from your heel to the top of your head, and from the palm of the hand on the floor to your fingertips stretching skyward.

Note: To treat scoliosis, do the pose on one side only—the convex side. *Do not* do the pose on both sides.

The Pose: Place a yoga mat's long side against a wall. If you are unsure of your balance, place a chair just off the mat in front of you and facing you.

Begin on all fours with the convex side of your lumbar curve closest to the wall. Carefully shift your weight onto the hand and foot of the convex side, raising the other arm and hand toward the ceiling. Adjust your support-

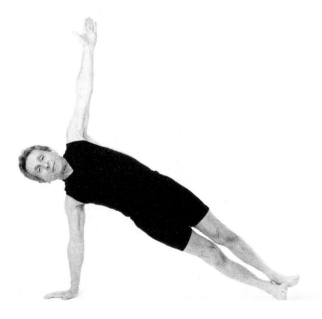

ing hand and foot so the arm is vertical and the fingers spread out, pointing slightly away from the wall. As you swing your torso upward, press both your shoulders and your entire back against the wall. Your upper foot should rest on the lower one. This is the time to stretch heel-to-head and across your chest from one outstretched arm to the other.

Now for the crucial addition that works against the scoliosis: raise the ribcage vertically as high as possible. That is, elevate the ribs that are closest to the mat on the convex side as much as possible. If this reverses the curve, making the upper side convex or bulging, so much the better. The final step is to keep yourself in this position for as long as you can. You must tire the muscles on the convex side in order to strengthen them maximally. You or a friend can feel the quadratus lumborum muscles while you're doing the pose to be sure you've got it right.

VARIATIONS:

There are many variations and modifications for people unable to perform this arduous pose. The chair in front of you can be used for balance, and can also help if the supporting shoulder is weak. Place the chair on your mat so that when you come into the pose, it is in front of your chest. Press your top hand into the chair for stability. Also, the foot of your upper leg can be brought forward to rest on the floor for stability. Either place your foot on its inner edge in front of the bottom foot, or bend your upper knee and place the foot flat on the floor, so that your thigh is at a right angle to the wall. Raise your ribs upward as high as possible in any case.

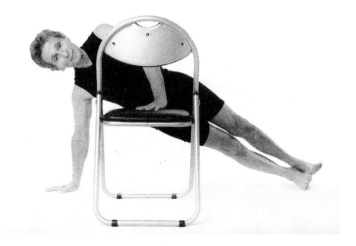

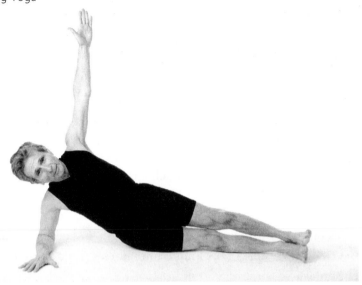

If you have carpal tunnel syndrome or Dupuytren's contracture, support yourself on the forearm of the lower arm rather than on the palm, and position your forearm at a right angle to the wall, palm down. If you don't have the strength to support yourself in the full pose, rest your bottom knee on the floor, rather than the outside of the foot. To make it even easier, support yourself on your forearm and hip. Again, lift the lower ribs skyward.

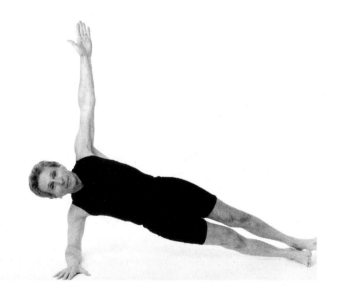

LEAST CHALLENGING VARIATION:

Lie on a mat or a bed with your back against the wall and do your best to raise the ribs toward the ceiling. Provided you stay close to the wall and align your shoulders vertically, even this pose will work, and soon you'll graduate to supporting yourself on your knees or hips and eventually possibly on your feet. With persistence you may proceed to the hand-supported version of the pose. The critical thing is to raise the lower ribs and torso away from the convex and toward the concave side.

Secondary Curves

Vasisthasana takes care of the vast majority of lumbar curves. However, the wisdom inherent in human upright physiology often makes for a compensatory curve higher up in the spine. Occasionally there is even a third curve, resembling the original one, but we will not talk much about it here.

If the lower curve is convex to the right, then the upper one curves to the left, and vice versa. Strengthening the muscles of the lower curve's convex side might have either of two effects on the upper curve: (1) since the concave side of the upper curve is on the convex side of the lower curve, the side that we're strengthening, Vasisthasana done on that side might worsen the upper curve! On the other hand, (2) once the lower curve's convex side muscles are strengthened and it straightens out a bit, that might reduce the tendency for the upper spine to curve, since there would be less for which to compensate.

So far, in my study, we have only seen the reduction in the lower curve bring about reduction in the upper curve, but the upper curve does not seem to get as much better as the lower curve. As the chart above plainly shows, in the few cases where a secondary curve was found, it did not improve as much as the primary curve, suggesting that both of these mechanisms were at work. Therefore, we have begun adapting Vasisthasana when there is a secondary curve, and we are working with another posture that seems to be more effective for the secondary curve without impairing, and actually enhancing, reduction of the primary curve.

If you have a secondary curve, you should wrap a belt around the midfoot of the upper leg in Vasisthasana, and raise it up away from the lower leg as much as possible with the thigh abductors, and then further abduct it by exerting strong, steady pressure on it with the free hand. Attempt to minimize elbow flexion by taking up as much slack as possible, but a perfectly straight elbow will likely be impossible. Do the pose once daily, and hold it as long as possible each time.

Ardha Chandrasana
Half Moon Pose

Some people have injuries that prevent them from supporting them-selves on the arm and hand in Vasisthasana (Side Plank Pose). Ardha Chandrasana, done on the *concave* side—the opposite side from the one we used in Vasisthasana—appears to be effective for them as well as for people with a secondary curve, though I have not yet studied it as closely as Vasisthasana. The short time in Triangle Pose does not seem to be harmful in any way.

Benefits and How It Works: Strengthens the convex side of the lumbar curve by supporting the torso from above. The pose also strengthens muscles located higher up the spine that are needed to reduce secondary curves on the opposite side.

Contraindications: Difficulty balancing, plantar fasciitis, vertebral fracture, Hill–Sachs deformity, subscapularis bursitis/tendinitis, subdeltoid bursitis, carpal tunnel syndrome.

Helpful Hints: Put your weight more on the little finger side of the supporting hand.

The Pose: Place your mat with the long edge against a wall. Stand with your feet three feet apart. Turn the foot on the concave side of your lumbar curve parallel to the wall. Turn the other foot 30 degrees in, toward the front foot. Stretch your arms out horizontally, as far out to the sides as you can. Take two breaths.

Bend your front knee so that it points over your toes and incline your torso over it. Rotate that side of your abdomen away from the thigh, widening the groin on that side. Reach down to the floor or to a block with the front leg's hand until at least the fingertips are firmly on it, approximately one foot

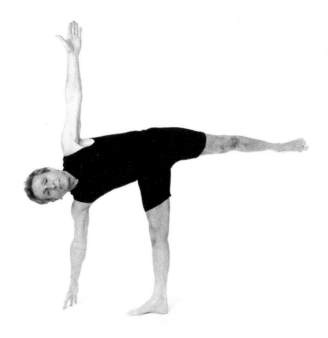

in front of the big toe and close to the wall. Now straighten the bent knee and raise the opposite leg up until the supporting leg is straight, and your torso and the opposite leg are horizontal. Your supporting hand should be directly below your shoulder. At first, rest your free hand on your hip and rotate the upper side of your torso until your upper shoulder is against the wall. As much as possible, gently press your back and the back of the horizontal leg against the wall. Straighten both legs. Stretch out from the heel of your horizontal leg to the top of your head, and across both arms. To improve your balance, put weight on the little finger of your supporting hand. Breathe slowly, fully and symmetrically. Whether you have a secondary curve or not, stretch the upper arm as high as possible.

To come out of the pose, bend the supporting leg and, at the same time, lower the other leg to the floor. Raise your torso back to vertical. If this is difficult, raise your hand off the floor and place it on your bent knee to help you rise.

Do not repeat this on the other side. The idea is to asymmetrically strengthen muscles of the bulging, but actually weaker side.

VARIATIONS:

If your major curve is convex to the left, place a chair at the right end of your mat, facing toward you. As you bend your right knee, place your right hand, or, if you have wrist or hand injury, align your forearm on the chair seat perpendicular to the wall. This variation has an advantage for people with secondary curves. After settling the right hand or forearm on the seat of the chair and entering into the pose as below, hold the underside of the seat of the chair with your right hand. Raise the left upper arm as far as possible, strengthening the convex side of the upper curve (the side closer to the floor).

I have used the pose pictured here to counter both parts of "S" curves effectively, and individual cases provide opportunities to use a variety of other poses and techniques.

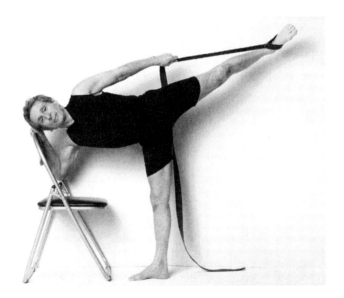

CHAPTER SIXTEEN

Premenstrual Syndrome

TIP

• Lie in bed with a heating pad on your
lower back or on your stomach.

• Don't eat pretzels, potato chips or other salty snacks
during the week before your period.

• Combine yoga with aerobic exercise.[1]

MANY EXPERTS BELIEVE that yoga can help women with premenstrual syndrome (PMS)—a group of symptoms connected to the menstrual cycle.[2] A woman who experiences symptoms beginning a week or so before her period and ending a few days after her period starts, and who has symptoms three months in a row, is said to have premenstrual syndrome.[3]

The standard medical definition of PMS includes a consistent pattern of physical and emotional symptoms, but we talk about it casually and we know what we mean without adhering to exact scientific guidelines. A woman who has even one symptom may refer to what she feels as PMS, which, until the 1980s, was widely considered to be another one of those conditions that was said (mostly by men) to exist in women's imaginations rather than in reality. Only then, partly because of the rise of feminism, was PMS accepted as a legitimate medical condition.

It is generally acknowledged that PMS is linked to hormone levels, particularly estrogen and progesterone, which vary as a woman's body prepares to menstruate. In my experience, there is a large range of PMS symptoms and those symptoms have large ranges of severity. For instance, a woman's low back pain may differ in intensity from month to month. In rare cases, PMS may be mistaken for dysmenorrhea (pain during menstruation that interferes with daily activities) or a bladder infection. But most experts think that more than three-quarters of women of childbearing age experience PMS symptoms not severe enough to interfere with their daily lives. In unusual cases, PMS can be so extreme that it causes huge upheavals in behavior. It has even been used as a criminal defense. Common symptoms of PMS are:

- Abdominal pain or cramping
- Bloating
- Low back pain and general aches and pains
- Swollen or tender breasts
- Weight gain due to fluid retention
- Mood swings, including depression, aggression and anxiety
- Anxiety
- Trouble concentrating
- Fatigue
- Irritability
- Food cravings
- Worsening of acne or appearance of cold sores

The majority of women who have PMS don't need medical care; they can cope with it themselves by controlling lifestyle choices and by using simple remedies. *The Merck Manual* recommends increasing protein, decreasing sugar and taking vitamin B complex (especially pyridoxine, vitamin B_6) or magnesium supplements (though it should be noted that magnesium can make one feel sleepy and has a laxative effect). Get enough, but not too much, sleep and exercise, and watch your alcohol and caffeine intake. When necessary, an over-the-counter pain and anti-inflammatory medication may be useful, especially a day or two before you think PMS might begin.

If you have severe symptoms, ruling out general systemic problems such as a thyroid condition is a good idea. After that, keeping a simple daily journal will shed light on what makes your symptoms worse. You can't prevent PMS, but you can get a handle on it. When you know, for example, that drinking coffee in the morning makes you feel worse during the days before your period begins, you can take action. I'm a believer in healthy eating and in all types of exercise, including swimming, and in taking a daily multivitamin. But for PMS symptoms such as anxiety, yoga can't be beat.[4]

Let me be more specific about PMS and yoga. Premenstrual syndrome has two main components: physical (cramping, bloating, headache, etc.) and emotional (lower self-esteem, sadness, reduced libido, etc.). Yoga, simply by being self-administered, helps you feel better about yourself. Clinical trials confirm that yoga helps reduce distress and depression and promotes a sense of calm well-being.[5] Check in other parts of this book—especially chapter 17, "Depression"—for poses that may help your emotional or behavioral symptoms. The poses that follow work to relieve the physical symptoms of PMS.

Paschimottanasana
Seated Forward Bend Pose

Benefits and How It Works: Can be done throughout the menstrual cycle. Reduces swelling of abdominal organs and tissues, calms irritability. The pose creates pressure in the abdominal cavity that squeezes out some of the fluid volume, where there is frequently swelling, and extends the volume of the retroperitoneal space, where ovaries and spinal roots are both located. It also prompts the pelvic diaphragm to relax.

Contraindications: Full stomach, vertebral compression or other fracture, -ostomies, ischial bursitis, herniated disc, severe hip arthritis, hamstring tear, osteoporosis (rare).

Helpful Hints: Contract the quadriceps, using the agonist–antagonist reflex to relax the hamstrings and gluteal musculature.

The Pose: Sit upright with legs together, knees straight. Bend forward from the lowest part of your hip sockets, drawing your entire body forward, not down. Use a belt around your feet if necessary (not pictured). Otherwise, hold your ankles or big toes, or clasp your hands behind the soles of your feet. It is advisable to work up to staying five minutes in this pose, breathing slowly, attempting, as Mr. Iyengar once said, "to make it as painless as possible," by enabling the muscles to cease contracting. Progressively use belt, hands on ankles, thumb and index finger grasping the big toes, interlocked hands behind feet, palms on soles, and finally one hand grasping the opposite wrist. Breathe softly, resting first the forehead, then the cheekbones and finally the chin farther and farther down on your shins.

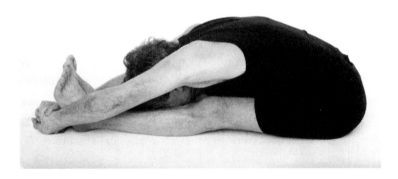

Ardha Baddha Padma Paschimottanasana
One-Legged Forward Bend in Half Lotus Pose

Benefits and How It Works: Improves circulation, especially drainage of the abdomen and pelvis, including the retroperitoneal space which houses the uterus, ovaries and fallopian tubes, as well as aiding drainage of the gastrointestinal tract, kidneys, spleen and muscular tissue of the abdomen.

This pose is similar to Paschimottanasana in that it stretches the retroperitoneal space that contains the kidneys and adrenal glands, the great blood vessels and lymphatic channels from the legs, and the paraspinal and related muscles. It is somewhat similar in putting pressure on the abdominal cavity itself, but does so more forcibly than Paschimottanasana both because of the lotus foot and because the pressure is being applied to only half the abdomen at a time, therefore doubling the pounds per square inch.

Contraindications: -ostomies, herniated nucleus pulposus, ischial bursitis, hamstring tear. Do not hunch forward. Use care if you have severe knee or hip arthritis, meniscal, ligamentous or labral tear, or total or partial knee replacement.

The Pose: Sit with both legs stretched out straight before you. Inhale and exhale as you bend the left knee and place the left foot into the right inguinal region in a half lotus position. Set both sit-bones against your blanket or mat, and straighten your spine. Address your two shoulders to the big toe and little toe sides of the right foot. Open your upper chest. Begin to bend forward from the lowest waist, aiming your head forward, not down. Aim your navel toward your inner thigh, your sternum toward your shin. Use a belt around the mid-arch of your right foot, if necessary, to retain the straight back as the angle of your forward bend gets more acute. Tighten the right quadriceps muscle as you descend, with your right foot vertical and perpendicular to the leg. Clasp your wrist behind the right foot tightly enough so the elbows do not touch the floor. Rest as much of the right side of your face as possible on the right shin. Breathe quietly but deeply for a full minute and enjoy the pose. Then repeat on the other side.

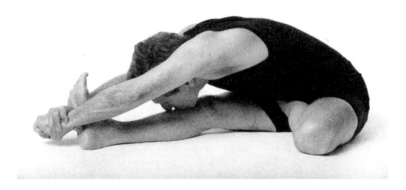

VARIATION:

Use a bolster, pillow or folded blanket on the thigh of the straight leg to exert more pressure on the abdomen and simultaneously help the lumbar spine and musculature to elongate safely.

Dhanurasana
Bow Pose

Benefits and How It Works: Reduces bloating, fatigue and abdominal pain.

Contraindications: Severe knee conditions, spinal stenosis, recent pelvic, lumbar or abdominal surgery, -ostomies. By simultaneously stretching the abdomen and increasing pressure there, fluid drainage is enhanced.

Helpful Hints: Breathe slowly, carefully and fully as you extend into the full pose. This pose may be done either lying face down or on your side. When done on one side it is known as Parsva Dhanurasana, which Mr. Iyengar describes as being the more difficult version. In the context of full-blown PMS, however, Parsva Dhanurasana, done with a modest or moderate effort, and props, is the sensible way to start. When PMS begins or even before it starts, the prone version may be more effective.

The Pose: Stretch out face down on a mat or blanket. Inhale as you bend your knees and lift your torso with your left hand and reach back to grasp your right ankle with your right hand. Then, supporting yourself on the arch made by the right arm and right leg, reach your left hand back and grasp your left ankle. As you breathe in this position, raise your torso and legs higher by releasing tension in your abdomen. Paradoxically, raising your legs higher will

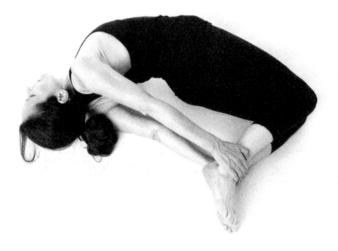

actually raise the shoulders higher by pulling the arms taut. When you reach a maximal elevation, adduct the thighs and calves together. First, stretch the head out far from your shoulders and elongate the entire spine, then raise your head. Breathing will necessarily be shallow, but continue to breathe calmly and as fully as is practical for 20–30 seconds.

You may also perform this pose on your right or left side, or both, as in the picture above. If you are lying on your left side, grasp your left ankle with your left hand first. Be aware of balance as a problem, and if inflexibility is a problem, use a belt hooked around both ankles.

Adho Mukha Virasana
Forward Bending Hero Pose

Benefits and How It Works: This is particularly useful for the back pain that may accompany PMS.

Contraindications: Severe kyphosis, osteoporosis (use pillows under the chest in each of these cases), severely osteoarthritic or post-surgery hips or knees (sit on blocks or pillows).

The Pose: Kneel and sit back on your haunches, using a pillow if necessary. Straighten your spine—get as tall as possible while making sure you are securely on your sit-bones. Slide your palms forward against the floor until your torso reaches your thighs. Draw your shoulderblades back, together and down toward your waist. Slide your palms far from your shoulders.

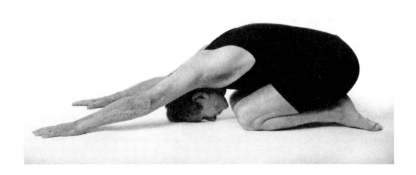

Uddiyana Bandha
Upward Flying Lock

Benefits and How It Works: Develops abdominal muscular control, coordinating it with movements of the head and trunk. By moving the abdominal organs, mild to moderate pressure is exerted on them, compressing out some of the excess fluid.

Contraindications: Full stomach, recent abdominal surgery, ventral hernia, -ostomies, abdominal arterial stents or organ transplants.

The Pose: Stand, inclined slightly forward, hands on bent knees. Lower your chin until it is cradled in the hollow below your Adam's apple. Take a deep breath and expel the air rapidly and completely. Hold your breath. Retract your entire abdomen toward the spine. Contract the anterior abdominal muscles and draw the entire abdominal contents up toward your ribcage and sternum as you press downward with both hands on your knees. With your chin down, holding your breath as you move your hands to your hips, gradually straighten your knees. This whole process should take about 10 seconds at most.

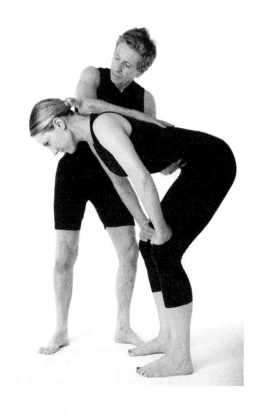

Learn it by doing it once daily for a week or two, and then do up to six or eight repetitions, but not more than one set per day. After a month or two of steady practice, you'll be ready to tackle Nauli. Although Uddiyana Bandha can be done all month long, Nauli should only be done when you are *not* having your period.

Nauli
Isolation of the Belly

Benefits and How It Works: Like Uddiyana Bandha, Nauli reduces menstrual cramps, bloating and other physical symptoms of PMS, but it is done in that part of your cycle when you are *not* having your period, as a preventative measure. By lowering pressure in the abdominal cavity, Nauli draws additional fluid to the region, prompting the lymph and other drainage systems to dilate and become more efficient so that when menstrual swelling arrives, the abdomen is better prepared to handle it. Also strengthens and brings better conscious control to the abdominus rectus muscles.

Contraindications: -ostomies, abdominal arterial stents or organ transplants.

Note: Nauli is a *kriya*, a cleaning process based on massage of the abdominal organs. A teacher or at least a video is often essential to get the hang of this.

The Kriya: Practice with an empty stomach after emptying your bladder and bowels. Stand, bent slightly forward, hands on bent knees. Lower your chin until it is cradled in the hollow below your Adam's apple. Take a deep breath and expel the air completely. Hold your breath. Pull in your abdomen back toward your spine. Now contract your diaphragm as though you are taking a breath in, but close the glottis so that no air actually passes into your chest. Your abdomen will hollow out dramatically as its contents rise. Hold that position for 5–10 seconds, not more, and then smoothly release your abdomen, and then release your hold on your throat, allowing air to enter your lungs. Do this once a day for a week or two, then gradually progress to three times during the day. After a month or two you will be ready to start the full Nauli.

The full Nauli begins as above, but after drawing your diaphragm down while holding the breath, do not straighten up. Rather, tighten the rectus abdominus muscle (the muscle that runs from the bottom of your sternum to your pubic bone), bringing it forward in your abdomen like a vertical band. Hold this for a few seconds. Release the abdominal muscles first, then release the hold on your breath. Continue doing this up to three times daily for a week or two. Then use the oblique abdominal muscles to create a wave of contraction, starting by contracting the muscles at the right edge of the abdomen and moving to the left, and then move the wave back from left to right. The idea is to bring these muscles forward in the abdomen by contracting them from right to left, then from left to right. Often this will prompt the hips to move rhythmically with the oscillations of the abdominal muscles. This is a natural and harmless thing.

It is best to do this up to three times early in the morning, after evacuating both bowel and bladder, before eating.

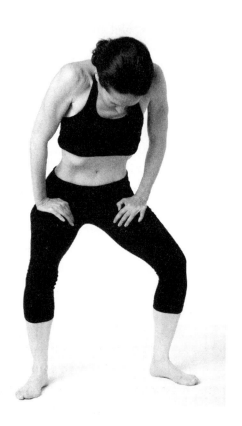

CHAPTER SEVENTEEN

Depression

I F YOU WATCH any television, you can't miss the ads for various antidepressant medications. No wonder: worldwide, more than 350 million people suffer from this mood disorder. According to the World Health Organization, depression results from a complex interaction of social, psychological and biological factors. There is a relationship between depression and physical health; for example, heart disease or chronic pain can lead to depression and vice versa, and people who are prone to depression have more physical ailments than those who do not. So many people have depression that you almost certainly know someone who gets low in the winter or at other times, or you may feel that way yourself.

There is more than one type of depression, and it can be related to age or life experience. For instance, up to one in five new mothers experiences postpartum depression. Nearly half of American college students report feeling symptoms of depression. Major depression lasts two or more weeks, and people who suffer one such bout are likely to have another. Like diabetes, depression requires long-term management.[1] Because of the stigma attached to depression, many people who experience it never receive any treatment. Yet many types of treatment, including yoga, can help enormously.

A depressed person often feels a sense of overwhelming sadness. Other symptoms include withdrawal from friends and family, fatigue, difficulty concentrating, loss of interest and pleasure in previously enjoyed activities, feelings of worthlessness and guilt, trouble sleeping or trouble staying awake, not eating enough or eating too much. A depressed person may express all this as anger or discouragement instead of typical sadness. There are all levels of severity to this condition, which can lead to suicide.[2] While the exact causes of depression are debated, it's suspected to have a genetic component and to be connected with the chemicals in the brain. Stress is a contributor. Depression is often accompanied by life events such as a death in the family, loss of a job, divorce or childhood abuse or neglect.

Non-Yoga Ways to Manage Depression

If you have depression that is more serious than a short-term mood change, there is a lot you can do for yourself, including yoga, which I will discuss in detail shortly. In addition to yoga, it will help to:

- Walk, swim, go to the gym, play sports or do any kind of physical exercise
- Structure your daily activities with a calendar or planner
- Don't try to take on too much; do a little less if you feel blue
- Eat a healthy diet; get enough sleep
- Volunteer or get involved in group activities
- Spend time with positive friends and family
- Read up on depression to empower yourself
- Limit stressful situations to the best of your ability

MEDICATION AND THERAPY

Psychotherapy and medication can relieve major depression, and they are particularly beneficial when used together. Cognitive behavioral therapy (CBT) helps patients to recognize and avoid triggers and to use specific, goal-oriented techniques for overcoming them. Group therapy is an excellent option for some. There is a host of medications for depression, some stronger and better than others, some with side effects such as weight gain and loss of interest in sex that make taking them unpleasant. Most medications take a few weeks to become effective, and it can take more than one try to figure out which, if any, are good for you. Some patients need a combination of medications.[3] My nephew, a family therapist, says that for many people who have depression, medication is necessary before talk therapy can become effective.

Yoga

Depression is a big, complicated subject, in which, for me, yoga is a central factor. The government database of medical journal articles lists dozens of studies of the use of yoga for depression. The studies are difficult to compare because of an apples-and-oranges situation: one clinical trial looks at the effectiveness of laughter yoga, while another examines alternate nostril breathing. Many studies include more than one modality—say, Pilates and yoga. But almost always, yoga is either definitely or probably helpful. I have not seen even one study that says yoga has a negative effect on depression.

Since Dr. Herbert Benson published *The Relaxation Response* in 1975, many illustrious researchers have duplicated his work and have gone further in investigating mind-body medicine. Transcendental Meditation, the kind that George Harrison and the Beatles practiced, was found to decrease blood pressure, heart rate and general metabolism, and to ease depression and alter cerebral activity. Dr. Benson identified two essential elements in the meditation process he studied. First, a practitioner finds a phrase that is either spoken softly or repeated to oneself. It can be almost anything: a prayer, a mantra, or a simple name are just three of innumerable examples. Secondly, you inhibit your mind from wandering, by simply turning your attention away from the thoughts, memories, plans or fantasies and calmly returning to the repetition. The reductions in heart rate and blood pressure—in fact, all the changes that Dr. Benson saw—were amply replicated, and the results of meditation and similar relaxation techniques are now reliably predictable.[4]

The beneficial effects of yoga for depression have been amply explored: for children and adults, for people who have cancer, for those with seasonal affective disorder and a host of other depressive problems. The Naval Medical Center in San Diego and other military and VA hospitals are offering yoga to help Marines, soldiers, sailors and others wounded in Iraq and Afghanistan who are suffering from post-traumatic stress disorder. Preliminary military studies have found that the calming effect of yoga can assist PTSD patients in dealing with hypervigilance, flashbacks, depression and anxiety.[5]

Key factors in the use of yoga to treat depression are that it's adaptable for the mood of the day or moment, and it can be done at home without supervision. Amy Weintraub, one of the most knowledgeable experts on yoga for depression, believes that it's important to practice yoga in keeping with your current mood. If you feel lethargic and have trouble getting out of bed in the morning, for example, a restorative back-bending pose with a simple breath practice helps to build energy so that you can get up and do the more dynamic and strengthening poses that are needed.

On the other hand, if you are suffering from anxiety-based depression (anxiety and depression occur together as much as 80 percent of the time), she says, "Beginning more dynamically can help burn off some excess energy." Amy suggests Sun Salutations or some standing poses to help with focus and clarity. After Sun Salutations, slowing down and adding forward-bending poses while extending the exhalation soothes anxiety.

In his book *Light on Yoga*, Mr. Iyengar lists the various illnesses that he believes respond to yoga.[6] Depression is not on that list, but fatigue, insomnia, loss of memory and "brain" do appear. For each of these conditions, he begins treatment options with Sirsasana, the headstand. While headstand is also recommended for other common medical conditions, such as rotator cuff syndrome (see Chapter 9), headstand puts things in a different perspective. Many people believe that headstand invigorates consciousness and heightens alertness. This may be because it activates many uncommonly accessed reflexes of balance and blood flow, including sympathetic arterial constriction in the lower extremities, and it partially reverses the blood distribution in the lungs so there is more blood in the upper lungs, where the air enters. To experienced yogis, it provides a familiar but changed viewpoint on the world. To newcomers it is that, and also a new source of confidence and independent accomplishment.

Sirsasana
Headstand

Benefits and How It Works: The pose initiates a different sense of your body, and therefore a different sense of yourself. Ludwig Wittgenstein alludes to this somatic sense of self when he writes "The human body is the best model of the soul." In addition, the pose is anti-depressant in the sense that your posture is not a slump or slouch, but firm and assertive, and thereby fosters that attitude.

Warning: Always use a blanket placed on the floor six inches from a wall to help prevent falling backward. Get the approval of a qualified teacher before doing head-stand without a wall behind you.

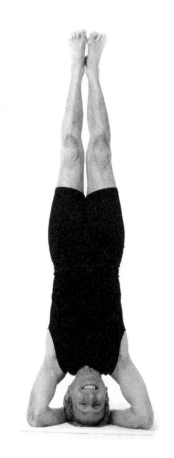

Contraindications: Imbalance, glaucoma, Chiari malformation, cerebral aneurysm or other cerebrovascular problems, herniated cervical disc, cervical facet syndrome, severe hypertension, orthostatic hypotension, history of head, neck or brain surgery, frozen shoulder, retinal detachment.

The Pose: Place a folded blanket on the floor with one edge against a wall. Kneel on the floor nine inches away from its edge. Clasp your hands firmly and rest them in the middle of the blanket to form two sides of an equilateral triangle.

Place the top of your head (not your forehead) in the middle of the triangle. Straighten your knees and slowly walk in toward your head, until your pelvis is over your arms and head. Then gradually lift your legs to vertical. Pull your lumbar spine back and advance your pelvis forward to arrange your ankles, hips, shoulders and ears as much in the same plane as possible. Use a mirror intermittently to establish this bodily integrity in the pose. After your balance is secure, press downward with your elbows and forearms and lift your shoulders far away from the floor. Keep your head on the blanket. Remain in this position for 45 seconds at first, though it is most effective in countering depression if you slowly build up to at least five and a half minutes.

Ujjayi Pranayama
Victorious Breath

Benefits and How It Works: This is a soothing but invigorating practice, analogous to taking a short swim in a peaceful lake on a warm day. It stimulates the parasympathetic nervous system, which promotes smoother functioning of the viscera.

The parasympathetic system has the opposite influence on the body from the sympathetic nervous system, which mounts the famous fight-or-flight or acute stress response. Ironically, Dr. Walter B. Cannon, who coined that phrase, did his work in the same room at Harvard that Dr. Herbert Benson used to delineate the relaxation response half a century later. Activating the parasympathetic system reduces anxiety generated by internal and external stimuli, which lightens the nervous system's load, helping the practitioner to relax. The amount of carbon dioxide in your bloodstream is generally decreased in Ujjayi, moderately reducing the impulse to breathe. This produces a heady sense of self-sufficiency that outlasts the changes in CO_2.

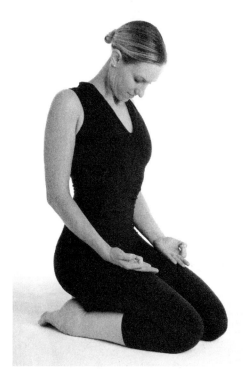

Contraindications: This is an extremely safe type of pranayama (control, or extension, of the breath)—possibly the safest. However, do not do it if you have hypertension; with well-managed hypertension it can be done lying down. Other contraindications are abdominal aortic aneurysm, cervical herniated disc, pulmonary hypertension or severe gastric reflux.

Helpful Hints: To practice Ujjayi, put your hands over your ears lightly. Inhale through the nose and exhale a whispered "ha" sound with your mouth open. After a few rounds, try producing the same sound with your mouth closed. When you're comfortable making the sound on the exhalation, try making it on the inhalation as well. Having your hands over your ears will help you focus on the sound of the breath—which is like the reassuring and comforting sound of the ocean. It is a very calming practice and can help soothe an anxious mind.

The Pose: Sit straight with your legs crossed, in any comfortable seat, or if you know how, sit in Padmasana (Lotus Pose). You can even sit in a chair. With spine erect, bend your head and neck forward to cradle your chin in the concave space between your collarbones. Hold your arms out straight. Gently press the tips of the index fingers against the tips of the thumbs in front of you, resting your forearms or wrists on your thighs. Close your eyes and focus your powers of observation inward. Inhale fully, filling the lungs from the bottom to the top. Expand the lungs, focusing on all sides: front, back, inside and outside. Do not bulge your abdomen out as you do this; instead, when the lungs expand toward each other, contract your anus and the muscles between it and your navel; draw your abdomen in toward your spine and up toward your liver and heart. Puff out your chest but do the opposite with your abdomen.

At the end of your inhalation, briefly hold your breath. When you exhale, use your tongue to guide the outgoing rush of air along the roof of your mouth. As you exhale, make a whispered "ha" sound and gently release your abdominal muscles. Repeat this series for several minutes at first, gradually working up to at least five minutes.

Meditation

Benefits and How It Works: The conceptual and emotional exercises that follow are intended to help you escape all the trappings that condition our experience and have a few moments or more of just being alert, not focusing on anything, not expecting or regretting, fearing or contemplating anything. The object of this is to promote perception of the vast inner silence, the cathedral of peace that subsists within each of us but which few of us have the opportunity to enter. It is a sure and simple refuge from depression.

Contraindications: None.

MEDITATION, THREE VARIATIONS:
Find a quiet place and assume a comfortable sitting posture, ideally with a backrest, and prepare to stay there, reasonably motionless, for ten to twenty

minutes. Let the backs of your hands rest on your thighs, look straight ahead and consider what you are leaving behind as you close your eyes.

WINDLESS PLACE:

Imagine a candle flame burning in a windless place. Ferociously hot, visibly responsive to any tiny breeze, but with all that combustion utterly still. Beautifully bright, full of activity but seemingly motionless. Let the flame, with its fixedness and its lightness, be a model for your own attention. Narrow it down to just the flame. Rest your attention easily and evenly on the flame.

Now comes the interesting part. Keep the focus but forget the flame.

ESTUARY:

Begin breathing in a slightly exaggerated way, either a little louder than naturally or a little deeper or faster. This already accomplishes half the task: getting your own attention. Gradually slow your breath and retain your focus on it. Then hold your breathing, but do not hold your breath; hold the act of taking in or letting out air.

Usually persons will close off their throats or use their tongues to obstruct their breathing passages while taking in or letting out air. You can actively create pressure with your diaphragm and the muscles of your chest, yet still no air will flow. This is what is commonly called holding your breath. What I'm suggesting is different. I'm asking you to leave all the airways completely open, and to inhibit action by the diaphragm and chest muscles. If a gnat were flying around in the room, it could go all the way down to the tiny air sacs in your lungs and zoom right out again without encountering any obstacle. This is what I mean by holding the breathing, not the breath.

This in itself will suspend your attention, and for a short time you will be focusing on nothing. In those few moments, broaden your attention so you are as alert as possible and as aware of as few things as possible.

It won't last. You will soon have thoughts, or memories, or plans, or emotional responses to things past, present or future. When that happens, lie down on your back, stretching your arms out, palms up, and extending your heels far from your hips. Again get still. Notice that breathing is something you can control, speeding it up or slowing it down. Next, relinquish all control over the respiratory process: do not consciously breathe; rather, let your physiology breathe you. Finally consider that breathing is an estuary between consciousness and involuntary reflex: if you want to, you can change it, but if you don't, automatic processes smoothly take over. Pay attention to this effortless, unmotivated act of breathing.

KICKING THE LADDER AWAY:

Focus on something that has been in your recent experience: a friend, a place, a planet. It can be something you like, don't like, or have no feelings about . . . anything. Think about it two ways: what it is like to know it, and what it would be like to be completely unaware of it. Finally, drop it easily from your consideration. The point is to generate enlivened interest in something and then keep the alertness without a specific object to absorb the curiosity—like climbing up a ladder to a hayloft and kicking the ladder away, and existing independently at the new elevation.

PART 5

Three Research Projects

As I write this today, things have changed enormously from the way they were when I began doing yoga as a young man, hoping to use what I had learned in my own practice and from my teacher, Mr. Iyengar, to help my patients get better. At that time people were suspicious of yoga, which seemed so foreign. It was something rock stars who also took drugs found interesting, something with mythology, like levitation, that seemed absurd. Most people would never have predicted that the number of those seriously practicing yoga and finding it beneficial would grow to over 20 million in the USA alone. Nor did we foresee that superb scientific researchers would be working diligently on hundreds of different studies, learning more about the way yoga works and what it can do.

The amount of clinical research being done excites me and gratifies me too, as nearly every day the newspapers publish a new study proving that yoga helps yet another mental or physical medical condition. The cultural differences between Eastern modalities and our Western medicine and attitudes don't seem to slow things down. The research engine is racing along toward many destinations. This investigation of yoga with scientific methods is deeply interesting and encourages hope for our green planet.

Treating patients every day, talking with the medical yoga therapists I work with about our patients and how to help them, and doing yoga with patients myself gives me ideas for more clinical trials, more investigation into different ways in which yoga might turn out to be useful.

Here are three poses and brief descriptions of their utility that I've begun investigating because I believe they have curative powers. Time will tell whether I'm correct in believing these poses might help, as the Triangular Forearm Support alleviates rotator cuff syndrome or Vasisthasana (Side Plank Pose) reduces the lumbar curve of scoliosis. As time and my practice of yoga go on, I'll probably have even more ideas. I certainly hope to continue to add to the ever-growing body of knowledge of medical yoga.

CHAPTER EIGHTEEN

Restless Legs Syndrome

This is a common problem affecting up to 10 percent of the population. Sufferers have their sleep disrupted by the urge to move their legs (or, less commonly, their arms); it can occur during the day as well. It has been characterized as a sensory-motor disorder of sleep/wake motor regulation that can negatively affect quality of life. Those with restless legs syndrome, also known as Willis–Ekborn disease, lie in bed quietly, waiting to fall asleep, when a buzzing or tingling in one or both legs irresistibly prompts them to move their legs, often barely readjusting them, at which time the vibrations abruptly stop, only to start again within a few seconds or minutes, with mounting intensity. No one really knows the cause of these distracting and recurrent symptoms. Some clinicians liken them to Parkinsonism, others to lower back disorders, and still others suggest that they are of unknown neurological origin, noting that sleep patterns in people with this condition have special characteristics. I'm in this third group, and it is because I was so baffled that I started to think not of discovering the cause of the condition, but simply of relieving it.

When restless legs syndrome is severe enough to send a person to the doctor, it is usually treated with dopamine agonists—medications that supplement dopamine levels in the brain.[1] It is fascinating to me that these medications work within the same neurological pathways as those that carry impulses from the brain to the rest of the body. They have side effects that include drowsiness, tremor, hallucinations, dizziness, impulsiveness and nausea.

Although these medications seem to be effective for many patients, a review article that looked at thirty-six clinical trials found that there was a 40 percent placebo effect—that is, a big percentage of patients got better taking a sham medication.[2] And, according to an opinion from the department of neurology at McGill University in Montreal, there isn't enough evidence to tell patients they can help themselves with changes in lifestyle, nutritional supplements or any specific nonpharmacological treatments.[3] Curiously, the dopamine pathways that are targeted by the medicines for restless legs syndrome are the same ones by which the placebo effect is believed to operate.

I'm not sure what the implications of that finding are for my method of treating restless legs syndrome with yoga, but I have seen yoga and yoga-like treatment bring good results. The movement inherent in yoga poses, like taking a long bike ride, may create an intervention large enough that the underlying conditions that brought on the restless leg phenomenon will change; the restless legs will become calm for a time, but the problem will return. What I came upon serendipitously is quite different, and has brought about total cure for quite a few patients. It is more closely related to meditation than to hatha yoga.

Overcoming the Difficulty
of Doing Nothing

Benefits and How It Works: Quieting of urges.

Contraindications: None.

The Method: In order to make best use of the treatment, it is helpful to review the general pattern of desire. In fact, this may be the most yogic part of the treatment. Desires, just about all of them, come in waves, beginning with an inkling, then a clear wish, then a full-blown urge that grows, and grows, and grows. If you watch carefully, the waves then start to diminish, then diminish further and further still, and then the urge is gone. The yogic treatment for restless legs syndrome consists of this observing. Just sit there or lie there and observe the urge to move and twitch grow and grow and then shrink, doing nothing about it. Don't allow yourself to give in. Then, after one or two comings and goings of the urge to move your limbs, after you have resisted once or twice, the urges will not come again. You might need to exercise this self-discipline more than once, but I have yet to see a case in which it did not vanquish restless legs syndrome.

You may need to build up to it. You might start by observing the growing desire to move your legs and, a few times, give in and do move them, which usually starts the cycle again. When you are ready, take on the challenge of, as a Buddhist might say, "not doing." You will be surprised, delighted and free of this disturbing condition.

CHAPTER NINETEEN

Bunion

Some Indian philosophers describe their ancient and fortunately vanishing caste system as like the three sections of the body: the priestly class is the head, the warrior, merchant and agricultural class makes up the abdomen and arms, and the group of people doing cleaning and unskilled tasks are the feet. "But the feet," the exegesis often continues, "are quite important." So is it with the lowly bunion, which can cause impressive pain and disability.

A bunion is a bony protrusion at the joint between the base of the big toe and the rest of the foot. Often, the big toe slants over in the direction of the other toes and is angled on the first metatarsal, the long bone that connects the toe to the mid-foot. Normal walking may put painful pressure on a bunion at every step, and shoes may rub on it or calluses develop. Contrary to popular belief, bunions are not caused only by wearing high-heeled shoes, though the squeezing of the foot and forward thrust of high heels certainly don't help. Bunions can be caused by arthritis, by having one leg that is longer than the other, by poor foot structure or by a genetic predisposition. Often there is no identifiable cause. This deformity of the foot, once it is full-blown, cannot easily be corrected. The medications prescribed for it give only temporary and partial relief. Surgery is just about the only recommended treatment, and though it is difficult, painful and involves a painful and lengthy recuperation of a painful month or two during which you really cannot walk, it does often work (though it sometimes worsens the situation).[1]

According to a clinical study done in Germany, nonsurgical treatment may relieve pain but will not correct the deformity. As far as I know, there has been little sound clinical research done on nonsurgical interventions for bunion, though there are claims that hinged splints worn both night and day can help.[2] My own yogic method is best begun early, when you think a bunion is developing. If you already have a large bulge, it will be more difficult to ameliorate with yoga.

The yoga treatment I think might have value is a single maneuver, with two parts. First you learn and practice the movement, strengthening and getting control over the muscle that is the foundation of it. Then you teach yourself to use the movement at the critical point in the gait cycle, as you walk.

Watching

Watch yourself walk. Each foot, as it starts to rise behind you, just before beginning to be brought forward to start the next stride, is supported by the big toe. Further, gravity pulls the outside part of that toe—the side away from the other toes—into the the ground or floor. Pressure against the outer part of the toe—the side away from the other toes—essentially pushes the big toe toward the other toes, promoting the formation of a bunion! This is a force we cannot escape; it is part of the process of walking on two feet. We cannot change the process, but we can invoke another, contrary process that is stronger.

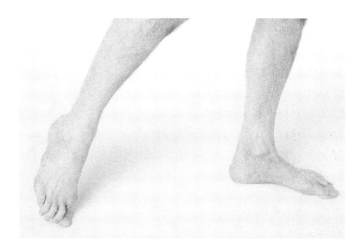

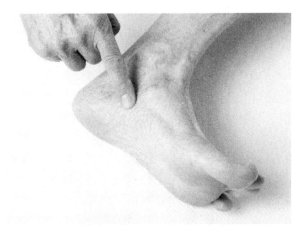

While standing or sitting, try to move the big toe away from the other four toes. There is a muscle—the abductor hallucis—that is in charge of that motion, but it is hard for some people to access it and contract it voluntarily. Work on it for, say, 20 seconds a day, when getting into the shower or at some other convenient time. Gradually you will learn to use that muscle and move the big toes 3–10 millimeters away from the other toes and toward each other. Be careful not to fool yourself by moving your feet; it is only the big toes that should move. Sometimes lifting the big toes up off the floor and extending them will help activate the abductor hallucis. This muscle is located on the inside of the foot, just above the arch, a little behind the medial malleolus (the jutting ankle bone). Put your finger on the muscle as you move the big toe outward to be sure you are contracting it. I estimate you need to do it 20–30 seconds a day for a month or so, until the muscle is strong and under your control.

When it is strong and you can contract it at will, you are ready for the second part of the treatment.

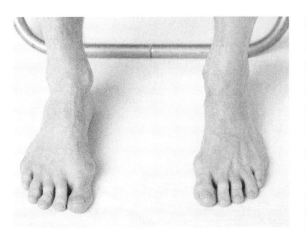
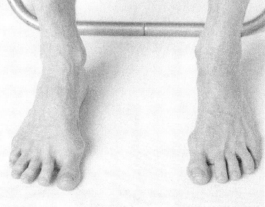

Opposing the Floor

The idea is to oppose the force from the floor that drives your big toe into the other four. Contract the abductor hallucis and press down on the floor with it when your foot is behind you and about to rise and move forward into the next step—where gravity is drawing it down toward the floor and when not much more than the toe is in contact with the floor. Contracting the muscle at that moment will oppose the bunion-creating situation, and in a number of cases I have seen, arrest its development and even reverse it. Sometimes the reversal is only partial, but in my experience if you keep up the pressing of the big toe into the floor just before raising the foot and starting the next step, you will keep the bunion at bay.

Use the muscle when walking a few steps barefoot in front of a mirror, then try a few steps with shoes on. Soon you will adjust to doing it naturally and unconsciously, the way you adjust to walking with a stone in your shoe. After a short time you will not have to think about it. After a longer time, possibly a year or more, I am fairly confident you will notice that your bunion is no worse, and possibly considerably better.

CHAPTER TWENTY

Plantar Fasciitis

Patients with foot pain, and particularly with heel pain, hobble in to see me nearly every day. For a long time their problem, plantar fasciitis, was conceptualized as an inflammation of the thick band of tissue that connects the heel to the toes and forms the arch. Now experts believe it is a weakening and tearing of this tissue.[1] Weak, ripped tissue can also cause inflammation, of course. A person who has this irritation of the plantar fascia experiences a sharp, stabbing pain in the heel or arch that is truly debilitating. The pain is worst in the morning, but it can last all day. It can appear after exercise, after being sedentary, even when climbing stairs.[2] There are all sorts of remedies for plantar fasciitis, but it is a pesky problem that often takes a long time—in my experience, up to a full year—to relieve. If you have it you can wear a heel cup, orthotics or various braces and casts, and you can try steroid and anaesthetic injections or have ultrasound waves driven into the heel.

Many runners and other athletes develop plantar fasciitis, and it often becomes chronic. People who are overweight, who must stand for long hours at their jobs or who wear improper shoes (including high heels and especially low heels) are also at risk. But one of the main reasons for the pain of plantar fasciitis is that the tissue covering the bones on the bottom of the foot is subjected to inordinate tension by strong forces dictated by the anatomy of the foot—for instance, flat feet, an arch that is too high, or gait abnormalities—accentuated by vigorous movement.

The reason the foot has an arch across its longer dimension and another that goes crosswise is to distribute the weight we bipeds put on it. Without the arch, all our weight would be concentrated just below the tibia and fibula, the shin bones. The highest part of the arch—the keystone, so to speak—is the navicular bone, which distributes our weight—and the forces we generate in running and jumping and dancing—to the heel and ball of the foot. But what holds the arch in place? Why is it not squashed down under this perpetual load?

A tough ligament, the plantar fascia, runs from the front of the foot to the calcaneus, the heel bone. Like a bowstring, it holds the bony constituents of the arch in a gentle but powerful curve. When you step on the foot, the bowstring tightens, pulling on its moorings at the forefoot and the heel. But even with the loads we carry and the games we play, the forces are usually insufficient to tear this tough ligament away from the bones.

So what forces are strong enough to disrupt this connection and cause plantar fasciitis? Our own muscles, those that flex the foot down to point the toe, and those that lift the front of the foot up if we were to walk on our heels, Charlie Chaplin style, are to blame. What seems to happen is that these two strong groups of antagonistic muscles fall out of their usual reciprocal reflex coordination and contract at the same time, pulling the front and back of the foot simultaneously, generating enough strain on the plantar fascia to rupture its inner part. Running and dancing do not cause plantar fasciitis. Rather, these activities strengthen the calf muscles sufficiently to tear the fascia with even relatively minor dyscoordination.

This observation—that it is our own muscles getting too tight at the wrong time—is behind the yoga treatment I have developed, which aims at stretching these antagonistic muscles and helping to recoordinate them.

Prasarita Padottanasana
Wide-Legged Standing Forward Bend Pose

Benefits and How It Works: Stretches plantar flexors and adductors. Lengthens the ankle flexors, thus reduces pressures on the plantar fascia.

Contraindications: Osteoporosis, recent herniated disc or ankle sprain, cerebral aneurysm.

Helpful Hints: Engage and attempt to relax the muscles between your gluteal muscles and your sphincters.

The Pose: Step your feet four and a half feet apart as you inhale, feet parallel, hands on your hips. Exhale as you bend forward at the hips, fingers forward. Inhale as you arch your back as much as possible, raising your shoulders and tipping your pelvis forward as far as you can from your hips. Take several moderately deep breaths. Then grasp your ankles and exhale as you gently draw your torso down into the plane defined by the intersection of your two legs. Be sure your whole torso moves, not just your shoulders and chest. Work especially with the inner thigh and leg muscles to stretch them.

LESS CHALLENGING VARIATION:

Rest your hands on two blocks placed in front of you on the floor, or use one block under your head in the second part of the pose, as you grasp your ankles.

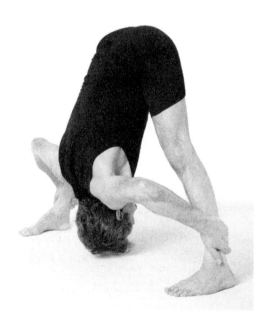

Trianga Mukhaikapada Paschimottanasana
Combination of Hero Pose and Forward Bend Pose

Benefits and How It Works: Stretches ankle flexors and extensors, and releases stress on the arches of both feet.

Contraindications: Severe osteoporosis, severe herniated disc, advanced knee pathology such as meniscal tears or cruciate ligamentous injuries, severe knee or hip arthritis or knee replacement.

Helpful Hints: Keep your back straight. Bring your torso forward; it will descend on its own.

The Pose: Sit to the inside of your left calf, left knee bent beneath you, right leg straight in front. Hold your right foot with both hands, exhaling as you draw your torso forward, navel to thigh, chin to shin. Remain in the pose for 30 seconds, breathing evenly. Then reverse the feet.

LESS CHALLENGING VARIATION:
Loop a belt around the mid-foot of the straight leg. Keep your back straight while you fold your entire torso forward, exhaling at the same time. You can hold the belt in both hands while drawing your navel toward the inner thigh of the straight leg. Take several slow breaths, then slowly release. Repeat on the other side.

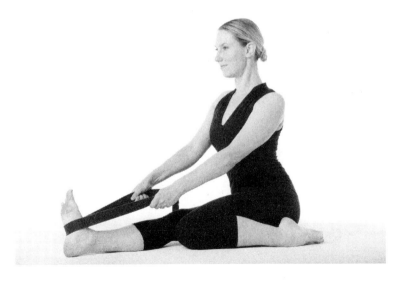

Krounchasana
Heron Pose

Benefits and How It Works: Like Trianga Mukhaikapada Paschimottanasana above, this pose emphasizes the alternate and reciprocal actions of the ankles, releasing stress on the arches of both feet.

Contraindications: Severe osteoporosis, severe herniated disc, extreme knee pathology such as meniscal or cruciate ligamentous tears, extreme knee or hip arthritis or knee replacement.

Helpful Hints: Keep your back straight. Bring your leg to your forehead, not vice versa.

The Pose: Sit to the inside of your left calf, left knee bent beneath you, right leg straight in front. You will naturally list to the left. Correct this by equalizing the weight on your sit-bones. Now bend your right knee and lift it. Hold your right foot with both hands, exhaling as you straighten and raise your right leg raise to your forehead or, better, your chin. Inhale to begin 30 seconds of smooth breathing in the pose; inhale again as you slowly lower the leg. Repeat on the other side.

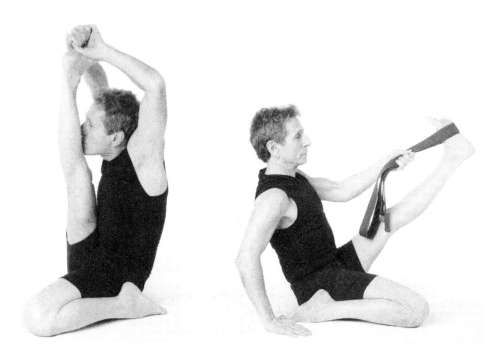

LESS CHALLENGING VARIATION:

Use a belt to hold the leg with the arm of the same side as you raise it to vertical. You can place the other hand on the floor or on a block beside the bent leg's thigh and use it for balance, or use a belt.

Virasana
Hero Pose

Benefits and How It Works: stretches knee extensors and ankle extensors.

Contraindications: Knee replacement or severe pathology such as meniscal tears, cruciate ligamentous or collateral ligamentous tears, advanced arthritis.

Helpful Hints: At first, use a cushion or two between your calves to remain comfortable when trying this pose. It can be dangerous if done without these props.

The Pose: Place two large pillows on the floor. Sit on the pillows, between your shins, after pulling the flesh of the back of the calves outward. Lengthen and straighten your spine. Place the backs of your hands on your thighs near your knees, elbows bent 60 degrees. Arch your back slightly and look forward.

As you become more comfortable in the pose, use fewer and smaller pillows until you are sitting with your ischial bones on the floor.

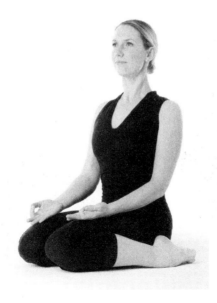

Janusirsasana
Head to Knee Pose

Benefits and How It Works: Stretches ankle flexors, knee flexors and hip extensors.

Contraindications: Osteoporosis, herniated disc. The temptations to hunch the back are great; improperly done, this is a formula for compression fracture and acute herniated disc.

Helpful Hints: It is better to go forward less far with a straight leg than to bend the leg, even if it seems you do not stretch as much. If the leg is truly straight, inhibitory reflexes are activated that relax the hamstrings after 30–60 seconds.

The Pose: Sit with your right leg stretched straight out before you. Bend your left knee and place your left heel high against the right inner thigh. Keeping your back straight, bring your torso forward. Hold your left foot, then hook your hands out beyond the side of the foot, clasping your left wrist with your right hand. Coax your chest forward, not down. Relax your elbows.

LESS CHALLENGING VARIATION:
Loop a belt around the sole of your foot. Remember to keep the back straight. Creep your hands forward along the belt until your elbows are straight. Even though you are descending, retain a strong back, as though you are holding the reins of a chariot. Aim the navel toward the front of the right thigh, rather than aiming your head toward your knee.

Other Poses for Plantar Fasciitis: Marichyasana I (p. 41), Ardha Baddha Padma Paschimottanasana (p. 192), and especially Parsvottanasana (p. 67).

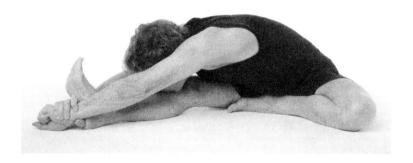

Acknowledgments

Thank you to Carol Ardman, coauthor with me of three earlier books; without her invaluable conceptual, analytic and creative editorial contributions, this book would not have been possible. To Suzanne Ausnit, for close reading and advice about yoga poses, and to Suzanne and Cathy Lily for invaluable help with the poses in the manuscript. To Tova Ovadia, whose physical therapy techniques and nimble mind helped me to create the TFS. To Megan Pederson, patient, persistent and smart manuscript helper. To Ellen Saltonstall, co-author with me of *Yoga for Osteoporosis* and *Yoga for Arthritis*, for knowledgeable contributions about yoga poses. And to my beloved yoga teacher B. K. S. Iyengar: he changed my life, and I thank him every day for the imperishable things he taught me.

Glossary

Abduction: The movement of a limb (or other part) away from the midline of the body. Opposite of adduction.

Adduction: Muscle moving a limb (or other part) toward the midline of the body or toward another part. The opposite of abduction.

Agonist–antagonist reflex: Muscles with opposite actions that inhibit each other. E.g., when the biceps contracts, the triceps relaxes involuntarily.

Anterior: Situated in the front of the body or nearer to the head; opposite of posterior.

Asana: Yoga posture.

Bisphosphonates (also called diphosphonates): A class of drugs used to prevent bone loss associated with osteoporosis, e.g., Fosamax.

Bunion: A painful swelling on the outer side of the joint of the big toe.

Cervicogenic: Coming from the cervical area—the part of the spine near the base of the skull. The place where cervicogenic headaches originate.

Cervical spine: The first seven vertebrae, generally denoted C1–C7.

Cobb method: A standard system of measuring curves of scoliosis.

Cognitive behavioral therapy (CBT): Psychotherapy focusing on changing negative thought patterns in order to correct negative behavior patterns and treat mood disorders such as depression.

Concave: Having an outline or surface that curves inward, like the interior of a circle or sphere. Opposite of convex.

Convex: Having an outline or surface curved like the exterior of a circle or sphere; opposite of concave.

CT (computerized tomography) Scan: Diagnostic test for bones and soft tissues; a series of X-rays taken from many different angles to create a cross-sectional image.

Dopamine: A small molecule manufactured by nerve cells as a neurotransmitter and a precursor of other neurologically active substances including norepinephrine.

Duodenum: The first part of the small intestine immediately beyond the stomach.

DEXA Scan: Dual energy X-ray absorptiometry: a means of measuring bone mineral density (BMD) with X-ray beams of differing (very low) energy levels.

EMG (electromyography): Nerve conduction test to diagnose neurological problems such as herniated disc, carpal tunnel syndrome, and piriformis syndrome.

Endogenous: Having an internal cause or origin: a substance made in the body.

Extension: The action of moving a limb from a bent to a straight position (e.g., elbow or knee extension), or toward the back of the body (shoulder or hip extension and arching the back itself).

Facet joints: Joints between one vertebra and the next that keep it in line, but allow it to bend and twist.

Flexion: The action of bending or the condition of being bent, especially the bending of a limb or joint or forward bending of the spine.

Golgi tendon organs: Tension-sensitive organs located in all tendons that relay information to the central nervous system and inhibit muscle contraction.

Hamstrings: Any of five muscles at the back of a person's upper leg.

Herniation: A condition in which part of a structure is displaced and protrudes through the wall containing it, especially a disc in the spine.

Hypertension: High blood pressure.

Ischial bursitis: Chronic and/or continuous irritation of the bursa at the sitting bone(s) in the buttock; often occurs in individuals with a sedentary lifestyle.

Kyphosis: Excessive outward (backward) curvature of the spine, causing hunching of the back, generally in the thoracic spine.

Ligament: Short band of tough, flexible, fibrous collagenous tissue that connects two bones, often holding a joint together. A membranous fold that supports an organ and keeps it in position.

Lordosis: Excessive inward (concave backward) curvature of the spine.

Lumbar spine: Relating to the lower part of the back. The usual five vertebrae are denoted L1–L5.

Mantra: A word or sound repeated to aid concentration during meditation.

Mesentery: A fold of the peritoneum that attaches the stomach, small intestine, pancreas, spleen and other organs to the posterior wall of the abdomen.

MRI (Magnetic Resonance Imaging): Diagnostic test that generates detailed three-dimensional images of the hard and soft tissues of the body, including muscle groups such as the rotator cuff and the nervous system, including the spine.

Neuroforamina: Spaces to the left and right of each vertebra through which nerve roots pass from the spinal cord to other parts of the body.

Osteoclasts: Cells that break down bone and return its minerals and protein to the systemic circulation.

Osteocytes: Cells that create bone.

Osteopathy: System of medicine originated by Dr. Andrew T. Stills in 1874 in the United States. Osteopathic physicians, known as DOs, as opposed to MDs, often use noninvasive manual and manipulative therapies and are known to focus on the "whole person." They are licensed to practice medicine and surgery in all fifty states.

Osteoporosis: Medical condition, frequently associated with hormonal changes, in which bones become weak and brittle because of loss of protein and minerals, especially calcium.

Osteopenia: Medical condition defined by reduced bone mass that is substantially less than normal but not as reduced as much as in osteoporosis. Osteopenic bone mineral density is 1–2.5 standard deviations below the mean value of women 25–30 years of age; osteoporosis is at least 2.5 standard deviations below that level.

Paraesthesia: An abnormal sensation, typically tingling or other sensations such as pins and needles, caused chiefly by pressure on or damage to peripheral nerves. Numbness is not feeling what is there; paraesthesia is feeling things that are not there.

Paraspinal muscles: Muscles running parallel to the spine which attach to it at both their ends; they provide support and originate many movements of the spine.

Physiatrist: A specialist in physical medicine and rehabilitation.

Piriformis muscle: Abductor and internal rotator of the flexed thigh, located in the buttock, in close relationship to where the sciatic nerve leaves the pelvis.

Piriformis syndrome: Painful condition involving compression or irritation of the sciatic nerve by the piriformis muscle.

Plantar fasciitis: Inflammation of the thick tissue connecting the heel to the forefoot.

Posterior: Further back in position; of or nearer the rear or hind end.

Props: Belts, blocks, blankets and other articles used to aid in doing yoga poses.

PTSD: Post-traumatic stress disorder, often associated with depression.

REM (rapid eye movement): A quick, repetitive motion of the eyes occurring in sleep. REM sleep occurs at intervals during the night and is associated with more dreaming and bodily movement, and faster pulse and breathing.

Quadratus lumborum: Powerful paired rectangular muscles connecting the lowest ribs to the posterior pelvis; a common origin of low back pain.

Quadriceps: Group of four muscles on the front of the thigh that extend the knee. One, the rectus femoris, crosses the groin.

Relaxation response: Physiologic changes discovered by Herbert Benson that include decreased activity of the sympathetic nervous system after stimulation of certain regions of the hypothalamus; can be self-induced through techniques such as breathing exercises, meditation and biofeedback.

Restless legs syndrome: Paraesthesia in one or both legs, usually occurring during rest, producing an almost irresistible urge to move the legs, at which time the paraesthesia stops temporarily, only to begin again within seconds or minutes.

Retroperitoneal space: Abdominal and pelvic space behind the compartment that encloses most of the intestines. It contains the kidneys, adrenal glands, ureters, pancreas (apart from the tail), spinal nerve roots, great blood vessels and the esophagus and ascending and descending colon.

Rotator cuff: The four muscles—supraspinatus, infraspinatus, subscapularis and teres minor—that facilitate and limit abduction, flexion, extension and rotation of the shoulder.

Sciatica: Neurologically caused pain along the course of the sciatic nerve that may manifest in the buttock, thigh, calf or foot.

Scoliosis: Abnormal lateral curvature of the spine.

Sleep apnea: Potentially lethal disorder in which breathing is significantly impaired during sleep.

Spontaneous fracture: Non-traumatic sudden fracture of a seemingly normal bone.

Stenosis: Abnormal narrowing.

Strain: Minor tendinous or muscular injury involving minimal anatomical alteration.

Sprain: Tension or torsion injury to ligament(s), causing rupture of some fibers.

Spasm: Prolonged involuntary muscular contraction.

Spondylolisthesis: Abnormal placement of a vertebra on the one below it. May be forward (anterolisthesis), backward (retrolisthesis) or to the side (lateral listhesis).

Stretch receptors: Neurological structures communicating muscular elongation to the central nervous system. Stretch receptors are present in all skeletal muscle and in smooth muscle such as the bladder, stomach and heart.

Subscapularis: A large triangular muscle of the rotator cuff that originates on the forward (anterior) aspect of the shoulderblade and attaches to the head of the humerus.

Subluxation: Significant joint displacement, (e.g., spondylolisthesis) less severe than complete dislocation but capable of causing pain and other symptoms.

Supraspinatus: A muscle in the rotator cuff that normally is active in abduction and flexion of the shoulder.

T score: A comparison of an individual's mineral bone density with healthy 25- to 30-year-old people of the same gender (USA) or with 30-year-old women (WHO).

Tensegrity: A structure held together by tension between its parts such as a tent or Roman arch.

Tendon: A flexible but inelastic cord of strong fibrous collagen tissue attaching a muscle to a bone, another muscle, or fascia.

Thoracic spine: Twelve vertebrae to which the ribs are attached that make up the middle segment of the vertebral column, between the cervical vertebrae and the lumbar vertebrae, denoted T1–T12.

Triangular Forearm Support (TFS): Yoga-based maneuver that clinical research has shown can reduce pain and disability caused by rotator cuff injury.

Ujjayi breathing: A yogic and Taoist technique for awareness and regulation which involves diaphragmatically drawing the breath in through both nostrils while partially closing the glottis.

Willis–Ekborn Disease: Restless legs syndrome.

Z score: The comparison of an individual's mineral bone density with that of an average person of the same age, gender, and ethnicity.

Sanskrit Pronunciation and Meaning Guide

The British were in India for hundreds of years, during which time they struggled with Sanskrit just as you may struggle to pronounce and understand the polysyllabic names of yoga poses. The English transliterations have become inconsistent over time, and alternate spellings exist. This promotes mispronunciation and a certain tolerance for different ways of saying these unfamiliar words.

Sanskrit, like German, builds larger words out of smaller ones. When you begin to recognize the smaller words (and I'll explain more about that in a moment), you will easily be able to sound out the syllables that make up the longer word. First, every pose name ends with the word *asana*, which means "pose" and like the word "fish" is both singular and plural. The pronunciation of that word is "ahs-a-na," with the stress on the first syllable and just a hint of the middle "a" as in "woman."

The letter "h" follows some consonants in ways unfamiliar to the English speaker. It generally indicates you should soften the vowel that follows it, which you can usually do by breathing out a little more than you otherwise would. One example is Salabhasana: "b" as in the word "better" (exhale a little extra), as'na." A salabh is a locust, and Salabhasana is the Locust Pose. You

235

can sound out Jathara Parivartanasana the same way: Jath, ara (aara), Pari (paari), vart (vaart), an (on), as'na, or Turning Belly Pose.

There is a wealth of information online, including YouTube videos and MP3 downloads, that can be found by searching "how to pronounce yoga poses." Here are some common root words for yoga poses.

Introductory Descriptive Words
Ardha: half
Utthita: risen or eminent
Parivrtta: revolved
Urdhva: upward
Adho: downward

Poses Named after Sages
Vasisthasana (t as in time; the h is silent)
Matsyendrasana

Poses Named after Animals
Kapotasana: Pigeon Pose
Gomukhasana: Cow Pose
Salabhasana: Locust Pose

Poses Named after Objects
Vrksasana (vriks-as'na): Tree Pose
Trikonasana: Triangle Pose
Ardha Chandrasana: Half Moon Pose
Setu Bandhasana: Bridge Pose

Poses Named after Body Parts
Janusirsasana (John-oo-sheersh-as'na): Head to Knee Pose
Paschimottanasana (posh-chi-mo-taan-as'na): Extreme Bend
    of the West Pose

About the Contributors

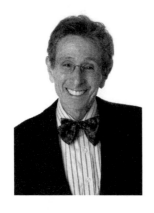

Loren Fishman, MD, a practicing physician who has done yoga daily for forty years, was described as "a Thomas Edison of yoga and medicine" by Pulitzer Prize–winning author William Broad, and has been interviewed on *ABC World News Tonight*. He received an advanced degree in philosophy from Oxford University, then spent a year with yoga master B. K. S. Iyengar in Pune, India, attending every class, public and private, and taking daily instruction. He attended Rush Presbyterian St. Luke's Medical School, did a Tufts–Harvard residency and was Chief Resident in Physical Medicine and Rehabilitation at the Albert Einstein College of Medicine. He is now on the staff at Columbia College of Physicians and Surgeons, treasurer of the Manhattan Institute for Cancer Research and medical director of Manhattan Physical Medicine and Rehabilitation in New York City, where he teaches yoga regularly to patients. He is a past president of the New York Society of Physical Medicine and Rehabilitation and has been one of *New York* magazine's "Best Doctors."

Dr. Fishman has written and edited more than eighty academic articles, chapters and books on rehabilitation medicine. The *New York Times* has featured his research, and his work has been reviewed in *Spine, Muscle and Nerve* and other international periodicals. He is currently associate editor of *Topics in Geriatric Rehabilitation*. Dr. Fishman's recent writings include *Yoga for Osteoporosis,* and *Yoga for Arthritis* (with Ellen Saltonstall).

Dr. Fishman was a featured speaker at the SYTAR conference of the International Association of Yoga Therapists in May 2013. He was awarded a prize for his research on a yoga maneuver to cure the pain and disability of rotator cuff tear at the First International Conference for Yoga and Social Reformation in Haridwar, India, in 2011. He has also published pioneering research on yoga for piriformis syndrome.

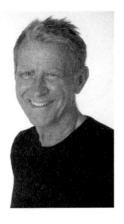

Chuck Baker knew he wanted to be a photographer at an early age. He received his first camera when he was in fourth grade, and by eighth grade he was working in a camera store. At sixteen—around the time John Kennedy was assassinated—he interned at the *Dallas Times Herald*. Chuck majored in photography and advertising design at Ohio University and then went to New York, where he became a photographer's assistant and then opened his own studio, Chuck Baker Photography. For years he contributed regularly to the *New York Times Magazine* and *New York* magazine, and worked for clients including Victoria's Secret and Ralph Lauren. Chuck still travels the world taking photographs of people, products and just about everything else.

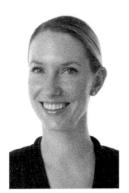

Lara Benusis is the manager of the Exercise and Yoga Program of the Integrative Medicine Service at Memorial Sloan–Kettering Cancer Center in New York City, where she serves on the research team and is featured in their online "yoga for cancer" teacher training. She is on the International Board of Advisors for Lohas International/Studio Yoggy, the largest wellness company in Japan, where she leads annual advanced teacher trainings.

In 2002 Lara founded and wrote the original curriculum for Children's Aid Society's yoga programs, developed the Namasteens approach and became the Director of Youth Programs at Pure Yoga NYC. She has been an invited lecturer for Quantia MD, Young Japanese

Breast Cancer Network, Survivors of Childhood Brain Tumors and NYU Medical School, and is a regular presenter at cancer survivor events. Since becoming a certified yoga instructor in 1996 she has taught over 20,000 hours, achieved dozens of advanced certifications, is a three-time international ambassador for Lululemon and is a certified ergonomic assessment specialist. She was introduced to yoga by her parents at an early age and plans to practice yoga for her entire life.

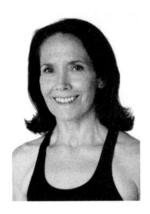

Cathy Lilly has specialized in training patients with injuries ranging from low back pain to osteoporosis with Dr. Fishman since 2008. She completed extensive yoga specialty trainings, including restorative, prenatal, postnatal, addiction, early Alzheimer's, cardiac, stroke and cancer issues, and is a member of the International Association of Yoga Therapists. Yoga was the primary method Cathy used in 2001 to become pain-free from her own lumbar herniation, cervical stenosis and rotator cuff injuries; these taught her what modifications help individuals with similar problems.

Cathy was a National Merit Scholar and was co-choreographer of and a member of the winning team of the NCAA National Collegiate Cheerleading Championship. Today she teaches group yoga classes and does private instruction and therapeutic yoga workshops throughout New York City. She is an expert source for the *New York Times* and has appeared on *ABC World News Tonight*. She is also an instructor at a yoga teacher training academy in Bangalore, India.

Notes

PART 1 BACK PAIN: An Overview

1 American Academy of Pain Medicine, "Facts and Figures on Pain," www. painmed.org/Workarea/DownloadAsset.aspx?id=3372 (accessed June 2013).

2 American Academy of Orthopaedic Surgeons, "Sprains and Strains: What's the Difference?" http://orthoinfo.aaos.org/topic.cfm?topic=A00111 (accessed June 2013).

3 National Institute of Arthritis and Musculoskeletal and Skin Diseases, "Handout on Health: Back Pain," http://www.niams.nih.gov/Health_Info/ Back?Pain/default.asp (accessed June 2013).

PART 3 NEUROLOGICAL BACK PAIN

Chapter 4 Sacroiliac Joint Derangement

1 S. P. Cohen, Y. Chen, et al., "Sacroiliac joint pain: a comprehensive review of epidemiology, diagnosis and treatment," *Expert Review of Neurotherapeutics* 13, no. 1 (January 2013): 99–116.

2 K. D. Christensen, "Rehab and the Sacroiliac Joint," *American Chiropractic Association Rehab Council*, www.ccptr.org/articles/rehab-and-the-sacroiliac-joint (accessed July 2013).

3 Mark Laslett, "Evidence-Based Diagnosis and Treatment of the Painful Sacroiliac Joint," *Journal of Manual and Manipulative Therapy* 16, no. 3 (2008): 142–52.

Chapter 5 **Herniated Disc**

1 US National Library of Medicine, "Herniated Disk: MedlinePlus Medical Encyclopedia," http://www.nlm.nih.gov/medlineplus/ency/article/000442.htm (accessed June 2013).

2 N. Henschke, C. G. Maher, K. M. Refshauge, et al., "Prognosis in patients with recent onset low back pain in Australian primary care: inception cohort study," *British Medical Journal* 337 (2008): a171.

Chapter 7 **Piriformis Syndrome**

1 Y. Yamakawa, A. Ito, and H. Sato, "Theta-toxin of Clostridium perfringens. I. Purification and some properties," *Biochimica et Biophysica Acta* 494, no. 2 (October 26, 1977): 301–13.

2 John D. Stewart, "The Piriformis Syndrome is Overdiagnosed," *Muscle & Nerve*, November 2003: 644–9.

3 L. M. Fishman, "Electrophysiologic evidence of piriformis syndrome," *Archives of Physical Medicine and Rehabilitation* 73, no. 4 (April 1992): 359–64.

4 Jane E. Brody, "Personal Health," *New York Times*, 15 April 1992.

5 Jane E. Brody, "Personal Health," *New York Times*, 12 January 1994.

6 A. G. Filler, J. Haynes, et al., "Sciatica of nondisc origin and piriformis syndrome: diagnosis by magnetic resonance neurography and interventional magnetic resonance imaging with outcome study of resulting treatment," *Journal of Neurosurgery: Spine* 2, no. 2 (February 2005): 99–115.

7 J. E. Kim and K. H. Kim, "Piriformis syndrome after percutaneous endoscopic lumbar discectomy via the posterolateral approach," *European Spine Journal* 20, no. 10 (October 2011): 1663–8.

8 G. J. Byeon and K. H. Kim, "Pirformis syndrome in knee osteoarthritis patients after wearing rocker bottom shoes," *Korean Journal of Pain* 24, no. 2 (June 2011): 93–9.

Chapter 8 **Combination Problems**

1 "Chronic Back Pain Shrinks 'Thinking Parts' of Brain," Northwestern University, November 23, 2004.

2 American Association of Neurological Surgeons, "Lumbar Spondylosis Sufferers Endure Lowest Quality-adjusted Life Year Health State Among Those

Affected by Common Chronic Diseases," *Newswise*, April 17, 2012, http://
www.newswise.com/articles/study-finds-lumbar-spondylosis-sufferers-
endure-lowest-quality-adjusted-life-year-health-state-among-those-affected-
by-common-chronic-diseases (accessed June 2013).

PART 4 INJURIES AND SYSTEMIC PROBLEMS

Chapter 9 **Rotator Cuff**

1   "Study Suggests Changes in Rotator Cuff Surgery Rehabilitation Needed,"
Newswise, July 13, 2013, http://www.newswise.com/articles/study-suggests-
changes-in-rotator-cuff-surgery-rehabilitation-needed (accessed July 2013).

2   M. J. Bey, C. D. Peltz, et al., "In vivo shoulder function after surgical repair
of torn rotator cuff: glenohumeral joint mechanics, shoulder strength, clinical outcomes, and their interaction," *American Journal of Sports Medicine* 39,
no. 10 (October 2011): 2117–29.

3   American Academy of Orthopaedic Surgeons, "Rotator Cuff Tears," http://
orthoinfo.aaos.org/topic.cfm?topic=A00064 (accessed July 2013).

4   S. Tempelhof, S. Rupp, et al., "Age-related prevalence of rotator cuff tears in
asymptomatic shoulders," *Journal of Shoulder and Elbow Surgery / American
Shoulder and Elbow Surgery* 8, no. 4 (1999): 296–9.

5   H. Razmjou, A. M. Davis, et al., "Disability and satisfaction after rotator cuff
decompression or repair: a sex and gender analysis," *BMC Musculoskeletal
Disorders* 12 (April 2011): 66.

6   Loren M. Fishman, Allen N. Wilkins, et al., "Yoga-Based Maneuver Effectively Treats Rotator Cuff Syndrome," *Topics in Geriatric Rehabilitation* 27,
no. 2 (April/June 2011): 151–61.

Chapter 10 **Headache**

1   H. Wahbeh, S. M. Elsas, et al., "Mind-body interventions: applications in
neurology," *Neurology* 70, no. 24 (June 2008): 2321–8.

2   B. Haque, K. M. Rahman, et al., "Precipitating and relieving factors of
migraine versus tension type headaches," *BMC Neurology* 25, no. 12 (August
2012): 82.

3   C. Wöber-Bingöl, "Triggers of migraine and tension-type headaches," *Handbook of Clinical Neurology* 97 (2010): 161–72.

4   National Headache Foundation, "Identifying Your Type of Headache," http://www.headaches.org/press/NHF_Press_Releases/2008-Press_ Releases/2008-04-Identifying_Your_Type_of_Headache (accessed July 2013).

5   The Complete Guide to Headache, "Headache Types: TENSION-TYPE," http://www.headaches.org/educational_modules/completeguide/tension2a. html (accessed July 2013).

6   R. G. Kaniecki, "Tension-type headache," *Continuum* 18, no. 4 (August 2012): 823–34.

7   D. C. Buse, A. N. Manack, et al., "Chronic Migraine Prevalence, Disability, and Sociodemographic Factors: Results From the American Migraine Prevalence and Prevention Study," *Headache* 52, no. 10 (June 2012): 1456–70.

8   D. Andress-Rothrock, W. King, et al., "An analysis of migraine triggers in a clinic-based population," *Headache* 50, no. 8 (September 2010): 1366–70.

9   N. Bogduk and J. Govind, "Cervicogenic headache: an assessment of the evidence on clinical diagnosis, invasive tests, and treatment," *The Lancet Neurology* 8, no. 10 (October 2009): 959–68.

Chapter 11 **Weight Control**

1   "Mom's Weight During Pregnancy Affects Her Daughter's Risk of Being Obese," *Science Daily*, July 5, 2009.

2   S. E. Berkow and N. Barnard, "Vegetarian diets and weight status," *Nutrition Reviews* 64, no. 4 (April 2006): 175–88.

3   OMICS Publishing Group, "Our Obesity Crisis Requires the Development of New, Widely Available Options: Can Yoga Function in a Major Role?" http:// www.omicsonline.org/2157-7595/2157-7595-1-e102.php?aid=1652%209 (accessed July 2013).

4   Adam M. Bernstein, Judi Bar, Jane Pernotto Ehrman, Mladen Golubic, and Michael F. Roizen, "Yoga in the Management of Overweight and Obesity," *American Journal of Lifestyle Medicine* 8, no. 1 (January/February 2014): 33–41.

Chapter 12 **Common Cold**

1   Society for General Microbiology, "Common Cold Virus Came From Birds About 200 Years Ago, Study Suggests," *ScienceDaily*, November 30, 2008,

available at: http://www.sciencedaily.com/releases/2008/11/081120073115. htm (accessed July 24, 2013).

2   Society for General Microbiology, "Common cold virus came from birds," *Alphagalileo Foundation,* http://www.alphagalileo.org/ViewItem. aspx?ItemId=1512&CultureCode=en (accessed July 2013).

3   F. Feuillet, B. Lina, et al., "Ten years of human metapneumovirus research," *Journal of Clinical Virology* 53, no. 2 (February 2012): 97–105.

4   A. L. De Sutter, M. L. van Driel, et al., "Oral antihistamine–decongestant–analgesic combinations for the common cold," *Cochrane Database of Systematic Reviews* 15 (February 2012): 2.

5   S. B. Mossad, M. L. Macknin, et al., "Zinc gluconate lozenges for treating the common cold. A randomized, double-blind, placebo-controlled study," *Annals of Internal Medicine* 125, no. 2 (July 15, 1996): 81–8.

6   Mayo Clinic, "Zinc: Dosing," http://www.mayoclinic.com/health/zinc/NS_ patient-zinc/DSECTION=dosing (accessed July 2013).

7   S. Qu, S. M. Olafsrud, L. A. Meza-Zepeda, and F. Saatcioglu, "Rapid Gene Expression Changes in Peripheral Blood Lymphocytes upon Practice of a Comprehensive Yoga Program," *PLoS ONE* 8, no. 4 (2013): e61910. Available at: doi:10.1371/journal.pone.0061910 (accessed July 2013).

Chapter 13 Bone Health

1   Health Physics Society, "In Memoriam: John R. Cameron," http://hps.org/ aboutthesociety/people/inmemoriam/JohnCameron.html (accessed June 2013).

2   US National Library of Medicine, "Osteoporosis," http://www.nlm.nih.gov/ medlineplus/osteoporosis.html (accessed June 2013).

3   E. Barrett-Connor, E. S. Siris, et al., "Osteoporosis and fracture risk in women of different ethnic groups," *Journal of Bone and Mineral Research* 20, no. 2 (February 2005): 185–94.

4   E. S. Siris, S. K. Brenneman, et al., "Predictive value of low BMD for 1-year fracture outcomes is similar for postmenopausal women ages 50–64 and 65 and older: Results from the National Osteoporosis Risk Assessment," *Journal of Bone and Mineral Research* 19, no. 8 (2004): 1215–20.

5   Man-Ying Wang, Shin-Yuan Yu, et al., "Biomechanical demands of therapeutic Hatha Yoga poses in older adults: Modified chair and downward facing dog," http://www.asbweb.org/conferences/2011/pdf/408.pdf (accessed June 2013).

6   A. Schmid, M. Van Puymbroeck, et al., "Group yoga intervention leads to

improved balance and balance self-efficacy after stroke," *BMC Complementary and Alternative Medicine* 12, supplement 1 (2012): 222.

7   Mayo Clinic, "Osteoporosis: Risk Factors," http://www.mayoclinic.com/health/osteoporosis/DS00128/DSECTION=risk-factors (accessed June 2013).   8   Harvard Medical School, "Update on osteoporosis drugs," http://www.health.harvard.edu/newsweek/Update_on_osteoporosis_drugs.htm (accessed June 2013).

9   Marcea Whitaker, Jia Guo, PhD, et al., "Perspective: Bisphosphonates for Osteoporosis—Where Do We Go from Here?" *New England Journal of Medicine* 366 (May 2012): 2048–51.

10 P. A. Howard, B. J. Barnes, et al., "Impact of bisphosphonates on the risk of atrial fibrillation," *American Journal of Cardiovascular Drugs* 10, no. 6 (2010): 359–67.

11 J. M. Fernandez-Real, M. Bullo, et al., "A Mediterranean diet enriched with olive oil is associated with higher serum total osteocalcin levels in elderly men at high cardiovascular risk," *Journal of Clinical Endocrinology and Metabolism* 97, no. 10 (October 2012): 3792–8.

12 Gina Kolata, "Healthy Women Advised Not to Take Calcium and Vitamin D to Prevent Fractures," *New York Times*, 12 June 2012.

13 Charles T. Price, Joshua R. Langford, et al., "Essential Nutrients for Bone Health and a Review of their Availability in the Average North American Diet," *Open Orthopaedics Journal* 6 (2012): 143–9.

14 Loren M. Fishman, "Yoga for Osteoporosis: A Pilot Study," *Topics in Geriatric Rehabilitation* 25, no. 3 (2009): 244–50.

15 National Osteoporosis Foundation, "I Have Osteoporosis. Can I Do Yoga Exercises Where I Bend at the Waist and Touch the Floor? Is It Safe to Twist from Side-to-side?", http://nof.org/faq (accessed July 2013).

16 L. Cristofolini, M. Nicola Brandolini, V. Danesi, M. M. Juszczyk, P. Erani, M. Viceconti. "Strain distribution in the lumbar vertebrae under different lading configurations." *Spine Journal* 13 (2013):1281–92.

Chapter 14 **Insomnia**

1   Thomas Roth, "Insomnia: Definition, Prevalence, Etiology, and Consequences," *Journal of Clinical Sleep Medicine* 3, supplement 5 (August 2007): S7–S10.

2   T. Roth and T. Roehrs, "Insomnia: Epidemiology, Characteristics, and Consequences," *Clinical Cornerstone* 5, no. 3 (2003): 5–15.

3   M. M. Ohayon and P. Lemoine, "Daytime consequences of insomnia complaints in the French general population," *L'Encephale* 30, no. 3 (May–June 2004): 222–7.

4   Alon Y. Avidan, "Epidemiology, Assessment, and Treatment of Insomnia in Elderly: Treatment of Insomnia in the Geriatric Patient," *Medscape,* http://www.medscape.org/viewarticle/516282_6 (accessed July 2013).

5   National Heart, Lung, and Blood Institute, "Your Guide to Healthy Sleep," http://www.nhlbi.nih.gov/health/public/sleep/healthy_sleep.pdf (accessed July 2013).

6   Consumer Reports Health and Best Buy Drugs, "Evaluating Newer Sleeping Pills Used to Treat Insomnia: Comparing Effectiveness, Safety, and Price," http://www.consumerreports.org/health/resources/pdf/best-buy-drugs/InsomniaUpdate-FINAL-July2008.pdf (accessed June 2013).

7   E. H. Kozasa, H. Hachul, et al., "Mind-body interventions for the treatment of insomnia: a review," *Revista Brasileira de Psiquiatria* 32, no. 4 (December 2010): 437–43.

8   D. M. Taibi and M. V. Vitiello, "A pilot study of gentle yoga for sleep disturbance in women with osteoarthritis," *Sleep Medicine* 12, no. 5 (May 2011): 512–7.

9   K. E. Innes and T. K. Selfe, "The Effects of a Gentle Yoga Program on Sleep, Mood, and Blood Pressure in Older Women with Restless Legs Syndrome (RLS): A Preliminary Randomized Controlled Trial," *Evidence-Based Complementary and Alternative Medicine* 2012 (2012), available at: http://dx.doi.org/10.1155/2012/294058.

10 Yogani, "Advanced Yoga Practices: Easy Lessons for Ecstatic Living," Nashville, TN: AYP Publishing, 2004.

Chapter 15 Scoliosis

1   P. De Baat, E. C. van Biezen, et al., "Scoliosis: review of types, aetiology, diagnostics, and treatment 1," *Ned Tijdschr Tandheelkd* 119, no. 10 (October 2012): 474–8.

2   Ibid.

3   B. Linker, "A dangerous curve: the role of history in America's scoliosis screening programs," *American Journal of Public Health* 102, no. 4 (April 2012): 606–16.

4   American Academy of Orthopaedic Surgeons, "Treatment Options for Sco-
    liosis: What Are the Treatment Options for Scoliosis?" http://orthoinfo.aaos.
    org/topic.cfm?topic=A00636 (accessed July 2013).

5   US National Library of Medicine and National Institutes of Health, "Lordo-
    sis," *Medline Plus*, www.nlm.nih.gov/medlineplus/ency/article/003278.htm
    (accessed July 2013).

6   S. Negrini, C. Fusco, et al., "Exercises reduce the progression rate of adoles-
    cent idiopathic scoliosis: Results of a comprehensive systematic review of the
    literature," *Italian Scientific Spine Institute* 30, no. 10 (2008): 772–85.

7   National Scoliosis Foundation, "Frequently Asked Questions," http://www.
    scoliosis.org/faq.php (accessed July 2013).

8   American Academy of Orthopaedic Surgeons, "Treatment Options for
    Scoliosis."

9   L. Rivett, A. Rothberg, et al., "The relationship between quality of life and
    compliance to a brace protocol in adolescents with idiopathic scoliosis: a com-
    parative study," *BMC Musculoskeletal Disorders* 14, no. 10 (January 2009): 5.

10 M. Ikai and T. Fukunaga, "Calculation of muscular strength per unit cross
    sectional area of human muscle by means of ultrasound measurement,"
    Int. Z Agnew Physiol. Arbeitsphysiol. 26 (1968L): 26–32; Y. Kunimune, Y.
    Harada, et al., "Recovery from exercise-induced desaturation in the para-
    spinal muscles in idiopathic scoliosis," *Spine* 24, no. 19 (October 1, 1999):
    2019–24; Z. Q. Chen, Y. F. Zhao, et al., "Factors affecting curve flexibility in
    skeletally immature and mature idiopathic scoliosis," *Journal of Orthopaedic
    Science* 16, no. 2 (March 2011): 133–8.

Chapter 16 **Premenstrual Syndrome**

1   Family Doctor, "Premenstrual Syndrome (PMS) Treatment," http://fami
    lydoctor.org/familydoctor/en/diseases-conditions/premenstrual-syndrome-
    pms/treatment.html (accessed July 2013).

2   "Premenstrual Syndrome (PMS): Menstrual Abnormalities: Merck Manual
    Professional," *Merck Manual for Health Care Professionals*, http://www.mer
    ckmanuals.com/professional/gynecology_and_obstetrics/menstrual_abno
    rmalities/premenstrual_syndrome_pms.html (accessed July 2013).

3   Womenshealth.gov, "Premenstrual Syndrome (PMS) Fact Sheet," http://
    www.womenshealth.gov/publications/our-publications/fact-sheet/premen
    strual-syndrome.html (accessed July 2013).

4   R. Nidhi, V. Padmalatha, et al., "Effect of holistic yoga program on anxiety symptoms in adolescent girls with polycystic ovarian syndrome: A randomized control trial," *International Journal of Yoga* 5, no. 2 (July 2012): 112–7.

5   A. Michalsen, M. Jeitler, et al., "Iyengar yoga for distressed women: a 3-armed randomized controlled trial," *Evidence-Based Complementary and Alternative Medicine* 2012 (2012), available at: http://dx.doi.org/10.1155/2012/408727 (accessed January 2014).

Chapter 17 Depression

1   World Health Organization, "Depression Is a Common Illness and People Suffering from Depression Need Support and Treatment," http://www.who.int/mediacentre/news/notes/2012/mental_health_day_20121009/en/ (accessed July 2013).

2   "Major depression; Unipolar depression; Major depressive disorder," *A.D.A.M. Medical Encyclopedia,* http://www.ncbi.nlm.nih.gov/pubmed health/PMH0001941 (accessed July 2013).

3   Mental Health America of Pikes Peak Region, "Ranking America's Mental Health: An Analysis of Depression Across the States," http://www.mental healthanswers.org/page.asp?pageid=0%7C164%7C178&id=0%7Cranking_america's_mental_health:_an_analysis_of_depression_across_the_states (accessed July 2013).

4   Manoj K. Bhasin, Jeffery A. Dusek, et al., "Relaxation Response Induces Temporal Transcriptome Changes in Energy Metabolism, Insulin Secretion and Inflammatory Pathways," *PLoS ONE* 8, no. 5 (2013): e62817.

5   Tony Perry, "Yoga Helping U.S. War Wounded from Iraq, Afghanistan," *Los Angeles Times*, June 17, 2013.

6   B. K. S. Iyengar, *Light on Yoga: Revised Edition* (New York: Schocken, 1979).

PART 5 THREE RESEARCH PROJECTS

Chapter 18 Restless Legs Syndrome

1   R. K. Bogan and J. A. Cheray, "Restless legs syndrome: A review of diagnosis and management in primary care," *Postgraduate Medical Journal* 125, no. 3 (May 2013): 99–111.

2   S. Fulda and T. C. Wetter, "Where dopamine meets opioids: a meta-analysis of the placebo effect in restless legs syndrome treatment studies," *Brain* 131,

part 4 (April 2008): 902–17; S. Rios Romenets and R. B. Postuma, "Treatment of Restless Legs Syndrome," *Current Treatment Options in Neurology* 15, no. 4 (August 2013): 396–409.

Chapter 19 **Bunion**

1   N. Wülker and F. Mittag, "The treatment of hallux valgus," *Deutsches Arzteblatt International* 109, no. 49 (December 2012): 857–67.
2   "Flexible, Hinged Split Corrects Bunions Without Surgery," *Newswise*, December 8, 2008, http://www.newswise.com/articles/flexible-hinged-splint-corrects-bunions-without-surgery (accessed July 2013).

Chapter 20 **Plantar Fasciitis**

1   Gretchen Reynolds. "No Consensus on a Common Cause of Foot Pain," *New York Times*, February 20, 2013.
2   US National Library of Medicine, "Plantar fasciitis," *A.D.A.M. Medical Encyclopedia*, last reviewed March 1, 2012, http://www.ncbi.nlm.nih.gov/pubmedhealth/PMH0004438/ (accessed July 2013).

Index of Poses by Chapter

Alphabetical Index of Poses